May Cause Side Effects

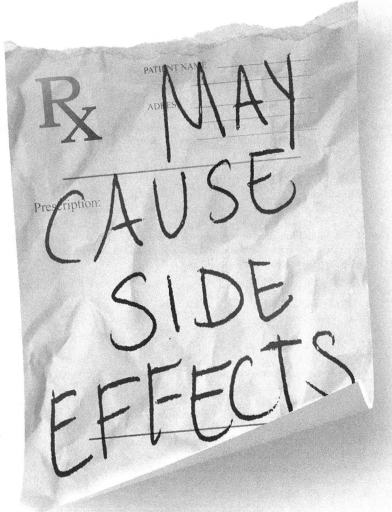

A Memoir

BROOKE SIEM

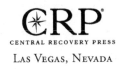

CENTRAL RECOVERY PRESS

Las Vegas, Nevada

Central Recovery Press (CRP) is committed to publishing exceptional materials addressing addiction treatment, recovery, and behavioral healthcare topics.

For more information, visit www.centralrecoverypress.com.

Publisher: Central Recovery Press
        3321 N. Buffalo Drive
        Las Vegas, NV 89129

28 27 26 25 24   1 2 3 4 5

Library of Congress Cataloging-in-Publication Data

Names: Siem, Brooke, author.
Title: May cause side effects : a memoir / Brooke Siem.
Identifiers: LCCN 2021055228 (print) | LCCN 2021055229 (ebook) | ISBN
   9781949481709 (hardcover) | ISBN 9781949481716 (ebook)
Subjects: LCSH: Siem, Brooke, Mental health. | Depressed
   persons--Biography. | Antidepressants--Side effects.
Classification: LCC RM332 .S54 2022 (print) | LCC RM332 (ebook) | DDC
   616.85/270092 [B]--dc23/eng/20211112
LC record available at https://lccn.loc.gov/2021055228
LC ebook record available at https://lccn.loc.gov/2021055229

Photo of Brooke Siem courtesy of David Goddard Photography.

Every attempt has been made to contact copyright holders. If copyright holders have not been properly acknowledged please contact us. Central Recovery Press will be happy to rectify the omission in future printings of this book.

Publisher's Note
Our books represent the experiences and opinions of their authors only. The information contained herein is not medical advice. This book is not an alternative to medical advice from your doctor or other professional healthcare provider.

Every effort has been made to ensure that events, institutions, and statistics presented in our books as facts are accurate and up-to-date. To protect their privacy, the names of some of the people, places, and institutions in this book may have been changed.

For Justin

Primum non nocere.
—Hippocrates

A Note from the Author

This book is not a substitute for medical advice, though it may help facilitate an open dialogue with your doctor. Never abruptly stop any psychiatric drug. Going off psychiatric medication should always be done under careful medical supervision. If you feel your health is being mismanaged, do not be afraid to seek out a different qualified professional.

introduction

There was a time—a long time—when I didn't believe I could ever be all right, that "all right" was a concept invented by whole people with whole hearts who could never understand how depression thumped inside me with the regularity of my own pulse. What did they know, anyway? Even the professionals told me I would never truly be all right. It was genetic, they said. Predisposed. A chemical imbalance. Like when a diabetic needs insulin. Take this pill. Come back in six months. We'll find a way to "manage" you.

It's no surprise, in retrospect, that ultimately this management tactic failed. I am not one to be managed, not even by selective serotonin-norepinephrine reuptake inhibitors, better known as prescription SNRI antidepressants. It was inevitable that the chemical tower I built around me would eventually crumble, given that I weaseled my way into the world in the presence of both a condom and a double dose of spermicide. Turns out I've been trumping pharmaceuticals since before I was a zygote. It's been my story all along.

Much ado is made about when a story begins and that story encodes itself into our bodies, quietly shifting our perception of the world. But the truth is we don't notice the start of our story. It begins when we are young and adjusting by fractions of degrees. The choices seem so free then, devoid of consequences and full of possibility. The choice to study this or that, to take the small job at the big firm or the big job at the small firm. To run. To rest. To love. To leave. It is only when we find ourselves in a psychiatrist's office ten, twenty, thirty years later that we realize how far off course we've strayed. At least that's how the story unfolded for me. Nearly a decade and a half after making a decision that seemed so small, so obvious at the time—to go on antidepressants at fifteen years old—I found myself staring at a patch of New York City sidewalk from thirty floors above, contemplating the biggest choice of all.

So this is where we begin.

I have intentionally left out many of the reasons why I found myself at that window, calculating the amount of time it would take to hit the ground. As a good friend once told me, "Pain is pain is pain." The details of my brand of emotional distress simply don't matter because there's no way to compare the depths of my pain to yours. We humans like to rationalize our way out of empathy by ranking emotional pain on a social scale of disturbing experiences (rape and murder at the top, finding out Santa isn't real at the bottom). All that really matters is that the pain existed. Besides, there are hundreds of other memoirs that can scratch the fucked-up-childhood-leads-to-mental-illness itch. This isn't one of them.

The reality is that suffering is not necessarily consistent with the severity of its origins. It is the reaction to the trauma that shapes our lives, not the trauma itself. If rational perspective could help us dig our way out of our own muck, happiness could be found in reveling in the fact that our problems aren't as troublesome as someone else's, and we would all be ecstatic. By that logic, even a guy living in a war zone with one leg blown off would be thrilled with his own life when he encountered some poor sap who was missing both legs! But we all know that's not how pain works. Pain is pain is pain. I am no exception.

Time has a way of warping our perception of the past. Throughout these pages, I've done my best to remain true to the narrative in the way it unfolded at the time. Other than changing a handful of names, the details I divulge are corroborated through journals I kept over the years, along with photos, emails, texts, tape recordings, and other people's recollections. But as with any human experience—especially one rooted in the mind—much of this story takes place in the depths of my psyche, which means you're going to have to take my word for it.

It must also be noted the topography of mental health is wide and full of landmines. There is no way for me to tell my story without running the risk of flipping an explosive switch. I cannot overstress how my story is just that—mine. My experience is but a single set of footprints on the sand, creating one of many paths for curious seekers to explore. I can tell you answers are not waiting at the end, that there is always more work to be done, and that it is only in the agonizing edges of ourselves that we find where our life's work lives.

It is in this place where true healing begins.

1

It happens like this:

It's December in New York City. I am at the window I've stood at so many times before. Only 5.58 seconds keep me from pushing out the rusted screen and bringing my body through. At 5' 3" and 125 lbs., with an air resistance of .24 meters per second squared, it would take me 5.58 seconds to fall from the thirtieth floor to the cement below. I know this because I count everything. Because I am clear in the numbers and clear in nothing else. Quantification brings order to the otherwise disorderly, lets me measure the immeasurable, know the unknowable. How many days until I take my final breath? I can't ever truly know. But I can curate an educated guess. I can take a dozen online life expectancy tests, sourced from retirement and life insurance websites. I can average the results and come up with a final life expectancy: eighty-three years, nine months, and five days for a total of 30,595 days on this planet. I can work a calendar, Leap days considered, and establish my day of death as November 6, 2069. I can schedule the event on my Google calendar at 12:00 p.m. on a Wednesday: DEAD.

I have been alive for twenty-nine years, ten months, and twenty-seven days. 10,922 days.

I have 19,673 days to go. It's a long time to wait to die. So I stand at the window. Wait for those 5.58 seconds to feel like relief. And tonight, compared to another 19,673 days, 5.58 seconds feels like freedom.

How easy it would be to go.

I walk to my desk drawer and grab a yellow legal pad. I'm not one for pithy notes and platitudes, so I write "19,673" across the page.

I cross it out and write "0."

How easy it would be to fall.

I close my eyes and count. *One one thousand. Two one thousand. Three one thousand. Four one thou . . .* nothing. Nothingness. Not like a blindfold. Not like sleep. More like trying to see out of your elbow. My mind can't comprehend the nihility and I want to ground it in something I can touch, something voluminous to quantify, to give this impossible weight a number I can point to and say, *See? It all makes sense now.* I don't have pebbles or pennies or grains or rice. Prescription drugs—those I have a lot of. White ones, purple ones, pink ones, gray ones. They mean something. They have a job. They calm the chaos. They right the wrong. They fix the broken.

I take my legal pad into my bathroom and open the medicine cabinet. Lined up in front of me, soldiers at attention:

Venlafaxine ER, brand name Effexor XR, 37.5mg, for depression.

Bupropion, brand name Wellbutrin XL, 150mg, for depression and anxiety.

Levothyroxine, brand name Synthroid, .05mg, for hypothyroidism.

Levothyroxine, brand name Synthroid, .075mg, for hypothyroidism.

Sucralfate, brand name Carafate, 1g, for bile reflux disease.

Isotretinoin, brand name Absorica, 30mg, for acne.

Ibuprofen, brand name Advil, 200mg, for daily headaches.

A generic multivitamin, for good health and wellness.

From age fifteen to thirty, this arsenal has varied in frequency and quantity, but not in kind. Only the isotretinoin is a newer addition, introduced three years ago in small-dose courses for a case of stubborn zits. The prescriptive party mix bottoms out at four pills per day and peaks at eight, depending on whether my headaches and bile reflux disease are raging. On average, I figure, I've taken six pills per day for a decade and a half.

I scratch the math into my legal pad, rounding out the weeks and years:

6 prescriptions a day x 7 days a week = 42 pills per week.

42 x 52 weeks in a year = 2,184 pills per year.

2,184 x 15 years = 32,760 pills.

I scribble 32,760 above the crossed-out 19,673. My entire life is tucked into those two numbers, one so much larger than the other. I wonder if 32,760 is a lot or a little in the grand scheme of a life and pour a day's worth of colorful allowances into my hand. They are light in my palm, a bit unwieldy all piled up one on the other. Until this moment, it has never occurred to me that I have taken three times as many pills as the number of days I have been alive.

I drop the capsules into the sink, go straight to the window, and press my forehead against the pane. The cold glass against my clammy skin calms the swirls of numbers in my mind. I can see Long Island City and Greenpoint glistening in the distance, as if the night sky descended onto Earth just to rest on the banks of the East River. Traffic backs up at the Midtown Tunnel. As the cars move, their brake lights crawl up the glass facades of the surrounding high-rises, illuminating the windows in spots of red and white. Sirens wail in the distance, caught somewhere along Third Avenue.

I open the window and examine the expanding wooden screen I bought during my first few weeks in New York. The wood is warped from eight years of rainstorms, blizzards, and blistering heat, and the mechanism to slide the screen wide or narrow is rusted shut. I struggle to dislodge the screen from where it sat for all those years and finally loosen it as an ambulance breaks through a wall of cars and barrels down the street in front of my building, only to get caught in traffic at the next stoplight.

Dangling the screen thirty floors above the sidewalk, I stick my torso out the window to get a good look at the stalled traffic. The ambulance screams for space, but it can't move. I wonder how many people die in Manhattan because the ambulance can't reach them in time, and how many more lose their minds as they watch their loved ones perish while sirens wail so close, but so far.

After 5.58 seconds, at least the ambulance won't have to rush.

A thought: *One third of those 32,760 medications are for my head. 10,920 antidepressants.*

The levothyroxine, the sucralfate, even the isotretinoin—they keep my physical body in working order. Right? But the Effexor and the Wellbutrin exist only for my mind, each orange prescription bottle a subconscious reminder that I Am Depressed and I Am Broken and I Need Fixing. Everything else is secondary. The loneliness, sadness, and melancholic hum of my life all validated by 10,000 antidepressants. I don't think about them when they get delivered to my door or when they slide down my throat. No doctor ever questions their use. No pharmacist refuses a refill. No lover lifts a morning eyebrow when he watches me from my bed, naked as I unscrew cap after cap.

I've been medicated half my life—and my entire adult life.

A gust of wind jostles the screen hanging from my hand.

And yet I am still just waiting to die.

How easy it would be to let it go. How easy it would be to watch it fall.

I have taken 10,920 antidepressants.

To let go. To fall.

Who might I be without them?

2

On November 6, 2069, exactly 19,655 days from today, I will be dead. Again. I have been dead many times before. Thousands of times.

I was dead this morning when I scribbled across a small, brown bag, covering up my bakery's logo before tipping a squealing, white mouse and its droppings out of a trap and into the crisp paper sack. I was dead when I stepped out of the bakery without a coat and into the blue winter sun, turning south on Clinton Street and hiding my face as I walked past my neighbors, hoping they didn't notice my bag of squealing contraband. I was dead when I ducked into an alley, crouched behind a beat-up, red sedan, and shook the mouse out behind the car.

"Go," I whispered to it, as it stood frozen on the icy pavement. I tapped its rump with the corner of the bag until the mouse found its footing and scampered away. Then I crumpled up the bag, hid it in a Styrofoam to-go box still wet with sauce, and perched the mousy evidence on top of a Manhattan trash heap.

I was dead eighteen months ago in a brownstone on 19th Street, trapped in therapy with my business partner, when our therapist deemed our relationship irreparable.

I was dead two years ago when, on the way to the bakery one early morning, a silver Honda T-boned the cab I was riding in. Out of the corner of my eye, the car came at me, and I wondered how hard it would have to hit for me to get the week off. I slid across the back seat, slammed into the side door, and scanned my body as shards of glass rained across my neck. *Not hard enough*, I thought, and climbed out the shattered window.

I was dead three years ago when I crawled into my mother's bed and curled up in a ball next to her. "What's the point of all this?" I asked.

"The point of what, honey?"

"Living."

She fell silent and turned onto her side, the two of us mirroring one another.

"Do you think maybe it has something to do with the antidepressants?" she asked. "Maybe they need to be changed?"

"My doctor said not to mess with them until things settle down," I said.

"You do have a lot going on right now."

"I think I was just born broken," I interrupted. "Like I showed up with faulty wiring."

"I don't believe it," she said.

"How can you not believe it?"

"Because this isn't the kid I brought home from the hospital."

"I'm not sure you're right about that," I said. Then I rolled off the bed and walked out of the room.

I was dead five years ago when I began baking out of my high-rise kitchen, lining every horizontal storage space in my Murray Hill apartment with rows of bite-sized cupcakes piped with swirls and finished with delicate mint leaves, cheddar crisps, and truffle salt.

I was dead eight years ago when I stood in the same apartment and nodded at my mother when she asked, "Are you sure, really sure, that this is the one?" I wanted the walk-up in the Village, the railroad-style apartment with dark wood, exposed brick, and a bedroom that barely fit a queen-sized mattress. But she needed me to be in a building with a doorman, she'd said the night before, tears filling her eyes as she squeezed my hand. "If you're going to be this far away, I just have to know someone is there. I have to. You're all I've got left."

I was dead twelve years ago when I arrived at Middlebury College in Vermont. Dead as I pretended to sip on warm, banana-piss beer in damp basements. Dead as I wondered how to relate to these Polo-clad undergrads who summered in the Hamptons and wintered in Wyoming ski cabins, when I grew up eating Christmas dinner at casino buffets in Reno and knew more about the legalities of prostitution in Nevada than I did about country clubs.

I was not yet dead fifteen years ago, somewhere off the coast of Italy, when my mother and I got the call. What started as a routine ulcer surgery was quickly thwarted when the surgeon discovered a grapefruit-sized mass of pancreatic cancer in my father's already bulbous belly. The doctors removed what they could and wheeled him out into a curtained room in the ICU, where he waited for two days, alone in a coma, while we traversed the globe as fast as air travel allowed. Naples. Frankfurt. San Francisco. Reno. Goodbye.

No, I was not yet dead when he died.

I am dead again tonight, but the wine feels cool against my throat. My little terrier mutt, Buffy, snoozes at my feet while I watch *Dateline*. *Dateline* is my reminder that even though I am dead, I am not *dead*. I need to dig through other people's pain in order to feel something, anything, even if all I feel is a twinge of morbid jealousy in between flashes of curiosity. *Dateline* cuts to a commercial for a class-action lawsuit. Something about weed killers and cancer. Hospital images fade in and out, victims attached to IVs while their heads hang in presumed medical debt. It takes me back half a life to the summer of 2001.

I was fifteen years old and standing in a hospital waiting room, peering through a small window into the ICU. Behind that window was chaos, a world of blood and bodies and endings, of tubes and gasps and force. A place where the difference between barely living and nearly dead was not a matter of will and love, but of machines and dumb luck.

"He will hear you," my mother said to me from across the waiting room. "His soul will hear you. Go."

A nurse took me through the heavy door and led me to the center of a large room, beds lined up next to one another like dominoes, separated only by curtains and ceiling rails. I scanned the room for my father's potbelly, the belly that peeked out between his usual outfit of worn undershirts and military Ranger panties, the belly I snuggled into while we watched scratchy episodes of *The Three Stooges* on beta tape. When the nurse shuffled through a clipboard of paperwork and led me forward to a figure, I thought she took me to the wrong person. Whatever was in front of me was not my father. My father was plump from cans of chili and sleeves of Saltines, his face sun-kissed from joyrides on his robin egg-blue Honda Gold Wing motorcycle. But all I saw was a sallow figure engulfed in a hospital gown, connected to miles of tubes and wires, belly deflated in the absence of a tumor.

"Take as much time as you need," the nurse said, closing the curtain.

I curled my toes in my flip-flops in order to keep my bare feet from accidentally touching the linoleum, suddenly aware I was in a hospital and the ground beneath me was diseased. My feet were still covered with a thin layer of Italian dust, gathered from the ashy village of Pompeii where thousands of souls perished under the blast of Mount Vesuvius in 79 A.D. I was wandering through the ruined ground just thirty-six hours ago, bodies entombed in final resting positions, mouths agape, fingers gnarled, eyes wide and waiting. A shiver had run down my spine despite the sweltering southern Italian heat. I could feel whatever *it* was that remained on Earth, the invisible ethers caught in each figure, frozen at the precise moment in between whatever this world is and whatever comes after. *They are still here*, I thought to myself. *Caught, held, imprisoned, the air is dusty and thick with them.* Now, I feel *them* here in the hospital, too. Caught. Held. Imprisoned by ventilators and dialysis and feeding tubes and false hope.

I stood over my father's yellowed body and examined the face for any signs of the man I knew, but his gray beard and the silver-rimmed bifocals that framed his ice-blue eyes were gone, replaced by hospital tape and bloat. His chest shook with each ventilated breath. A heart monitor beeped with obligation. It seemed silly to speak to this figure as if it was something I recognized. What do you say to the match before it lights the house on fire?

"Hi, Dad," I murmured, too self-conscious to speak. A part of me waited for his response, but the rest of me knew he wouldn't ever talk again. Still, I took his hand and waited for him to squeeze it back, to give me any indication he could hear me like my mother said he would. His hand stayed balmy and still, yet his cuticles, I noticed, were smooth. For all my life, I watched him chew at his cuticles until they bled. The wet smack of his lips around his fingers drove me nuts. The last time I saw him, I knocked his hand out of his mouth while he carpooled me to my first driver's ed class. "Most people look at the car in front of them," he said, gnawing at his thumb in between gestures toward a swerving clunker right in front of us. "You need to be looking five or six cars ahead to know what's going on with traffic. If that piece of shit Oldsmobile suddenly stops, you won't have time to react. If you're looking ahead, you'll see a problem in time to get the hell out of the way." He began chewing on his cuticle again. I reached across the car and slapped his hand away. This hand. The one on top of the hospital sheets. The one held in mine.

On the other side of the curtain I heard doctor chatter, the shuffle of documents, the squeak of a rusty wheel. I placed his hand back on the bed, his once mangled fingers now resting gray and shiny, and wondered how much time was the right amount of time to say goodbye. Does simply standing next to someone while they die even count as saying goodbye?

I didn't cry for weeks. I didn't cry at the memorial service, packed shoulder to sweaty shoulder into an old barn on the outskirts of Reno. I didn't cry when the barn doors flew open and a dozen of my father's motorcycle buddies revved their Harleys in a howling display of honor and grief. I didn't cry when my father's best friend, Darrel, went up to the microphone and told the story of how my father wrote a letter to Senator Harry Reid after Reid weighed in on a proposed Nevada law that would outlaw concealed weapons for citizens but exempted local, state, and national politicians. The letter began:

> Hey, Harry asshole, where do you think you're living, in New York? In case you haven't noticed, we live in Nevada, the Wild West, where law-abiding citizens have rights and firearms. And thanks for your bullshit letter on Healthcare. I told you I was watching your voting record. Between the two issues, you leave me no other choice but to vote for anyone other than you when your term expires. How can I and Nevada do any worse?

"Had Warren stopped there," Darrel said, "perhaps his little letter wouldn't have ended up with the FBI. But in full I-don't-give-a-shit mode, he concluded the letter with the comforting postscript: 'Hug your gun. You'll need it.'"

The barn erupted in laughter. It was standing room only, filled with people I didn't know from the parts of my father's life that existed outside of me. For hours, people told stories. In between each one, the crowd's mumbles slowed to a whisper. Soon, only the sound of a tissue box passing from person to person lingered. I sat with my back to them, feeling their eyeballs dart from my mother to me.

Do not cry, I commanded to myself in the silence. *That's what they expect you to do.*

My mother took my hand and squeezed it. I squeezed back and a flood of tears welled up in her eyes.

Do not cry. Be her rock.

I looked to a dusty piano sitting a few feet away from me. There was only one song to play, "Watermark" by Enya, an instrumental arrangement in F major featuring symphonic synthesizers and ethereal piano. Each time someone finished at the microphone, I thought about walking to the piano and playing the song, the song my father always asked me to play. But something held me back. Despite their stories and memories, they didn't really know him.

They didn't know he was so dyslexic he read the newspaper upside down. They didn't know he always wanted to learn to play the harp, but his fat fingers fumbled on the strings. They didn't know he was colorblind and earned the nickname "Unabomber" thanks to his distaste for societal norms and a wardrobe that primarily included black Velcro shoes and an assortment of deep-purple sweat suits.

They didn't know he slept at odd hours and snored like a freight train. On the days when insomnia got the best of him or he woke up at two in the morning after going to bed before dinner, he wandered downstairs naked, hoping for an off-season Easter egg hunt planted by my mother. She hid candies in bookshelves and under cushions, and he thumped about looking for his treasure. On the nights when she hadn't hidden little chocolate eggs around the house, my father went into the garage and sat in our brown sedan, bare-assed with the seat warmer turned to high, munching on a Costco-sized bag of Starbursts while blasting Enya through the car speakers.

They didn't know he was once suicidal, but that a therapist told him if he went through with taking his own life, he would ruin mine. According to my mother, "He never brought it up again."

They didn't know about his endless trough of rage that sent metal garbage cans flying into walls and computers smashing into the ground. They didn't know he once got so angry he threw a hammer into a fireplace mantle, only to have it ricochet right back into his front teeth. They didn't know he brought me smashed keyboards along with a screwdriver and a soldering iron and taught me how to piece the things back together. They didn't know that when he smiled, his front three teeth were fake.

They didn't know how loud he was, but on the day he walked out of our house with a loaded shotgun to right a perceived wrong, it was the quietest he'd ever been. My mother stopped him before he got to the car, but said, "His silence was booming. I could feel it in my soul."

They didn't know he never wanted children, and that the summer my mother found out she was pregnant with me, my father tried to cause a miscarriage by bouncing her in a speedboat on a stormy day.

But he changed. He honest-to-God *changed*. Once I got older and could walk and talk and learn, he came around. He took me to daddy-daughter dances, volunteered at my school every week, led group camping trips. We spent every weekend together in our mountain cabin, just the two of us. He taught me to shovel snow and build model trains and fix a broken toilet. He still threw fits and put his fists through walls, but his rage was never directed at me. Did I ever feel unloved or unsafe? Not once.

"Watermark" was his anthem. When the track came on while we were in the car together, it soothed his rough edges, quieting his string of expletives toward idiot drivers and calming him enough to release his cuticles from the clamp of his teeth. He turned up the volume and stopped talking until the last note faded away and for two minutes and twenty-two seconds, we found peace. I learned to play the song just for him, to create peace in our home as well. When his fits shook the entire house I went to the piano and played. My father would emerge from whatever corner he was in, close his eyes, and listen. The music spoke to the gentle depths of him that he so rarely revealed to anyone but me. It was our heart song, our language, our eternal connection. And though a part of me wanted to pound the barn's piano on that sizzling July day and let the notes rise up to join whatever soul was left of him, I also knew no one else would understand what the music meant.

So I left the keys unplayed. But in between each eulogy, as I waited for another story to be told, I tapped my fingers across my lap: F, C, G, A, G, C. The notes lived in my bones.

I didn't cry when we scattered his ashes under an evergreen tree with its branches all catawampus at the top, a quirk that reminded my mother and me of my father's bedhead. I didn't cry when I got my learner's permit and took my father's beloved, silver sports car out for a 100-mph joyride, days before my mother sold the car. I didn't cry on a Tuesday morning in September, when I turned on the TV to find one half of the World Trade Center on fire, a single matchstick burning on the small screen. I didn't cry when the weight of humanity seemed to sprinkle over my fifteen-year-old shoulders as the North Tower fell. Loss is loss is loss. No matter the circumstance.

I didn't cry when my mother and I both shrunk into five-feet-tall figures of hips and bones, subsisting on nothing but deviled eggs my grandmother delivered by the dozen. I wanted to run to my mother. And run away from her. I wanted to press fast forward or rewind and send us forward or back; it didn't matter as long as we weren't there. When I saw my mother's red and swollen eyes, I knew I was powerless to help her. So we danced around each other, co-existing in a haze of involuntary life. Sometimes my mother slept all day and sometimes she didn't sleep at all. Sometimes we hugged each other in the hallway. Sometimes we didn't acknowledge each other. Mostly, she was out of the house dealing with the logistics of sudden death. My parents owned a small company together, so my mother didn't just have to manage the loss of a husband, but a business partner, too. When she went through my father's office, she found a stack of recently organized folders containing documents, account numbers, and passwords only my father knew. She wondered if he knew he was sick, but didn't tell her. I didn't cry when she asked me what I thought. It didn't seem to matter either way.

I didn't cry until one fall afternoon, when I pulled a knife out of my flesh. It bored so deep into the fleshy space between my thumb and forefinger, that when I lifted my hand from the apple I'd been steadying, the knife held its place like a sixth appendage. I looked at my polydactyl hand for a few moments, perplexed because I felt no pain. When I grabbed the wooden handle and yanked, no blood appeared, so I steadied the apple again and went in for a slice.

Then it came, pouring out from deep within the centimeter gash, falling down my forearm, and soaking the half-cut apple. I grabbed the nearest dish towel and held my hand over the sink. When I lifted up the towel to check the wound, blood erupted like magma finally released after eons trapped by the pressure of Earth. By the time I picked up the phone to call my mother at the office and insist she come home, the dish towel was slick with red.

My mother found me fifteen minutes later, curled over the sink, sobbing into a puddle of blood. I howled as she wrapped my hand in a new towel and led me to the car. The wound was narrow, but the cut went deep. When I looked at it on the way to the urgent care, my mother had to pull over to let me throw up on the curb. I threw up again in the waiting room, and the nurses carted me away because my hysterics disturbed the rest of the patients.

"I'm going to need her to calm down," the doctor said to my mother as he handed me a barf bag and prepared to stitch me up. "It's only one stitch. I don't understand what the problem is."

I turned my head away from him and continued to sob, embarrassed and unable to catch my breath or hold still. A nurse caught my eye and glared at me while she washed her hands, organized boxes of gloves, and scribbled across my chart.

"Her father just died," my mother snapped. "It's not about the stitch. She's fifteen. Give her a damn break."

The doctor adjusted his glasses, grabbed my bloody hand, and muttered in a softened voice, "I'm sorry to hear that. I promise I can do this quickly, but you have to relax."

He slid the suture through my skin, fusing the severed flesh back together again. I felt the wiry thread pull deep within me as he tied a single knot, willing myself to be less space while my mother held my good hand, tears filling her eyes as she whispered, "I know, honey, I know. It's okay. It's okay." I kept still, wishing I could disappear from the impatient doctor, the leer of the nurse, and the heartbreak of my mother. When the doctor snipped the stitch and backed away, I gasped for breath, then puked.

The scar was still thick and tender a few months later. I ran my fingertips across it during my first appointment with Dr. Sanders, a child psychologist my mother insisted I see. She was a pale and plump woman who, against her office's mahogany floors, struck me as a polyp invading deep, rich skin. I wanted to scratch her out of my existence before she opened her mouth. I was a teenager with the internet. I knew from before I set foot in her office that I was dating anorexia and having the occasional affair with bulimia. I was ripe for a clinical diagnosis.

I also knew that even if I whittled down forty pounds of skin and bones, I would still take up space. Even in death, I would take up space, either in the form of a six-foot-by-four-foot plot of land or in ashes stuffed into a twelve-inch-by-eight-inch pine box that would live in the closet right next to the twelve-by-eight box that contained all the space that was once my father. No amount of shrinking could erase the space.

So I talked.

"I think I have an eating disorder," I told her.

"Why do you think that?" Dr. Sanders asked.

I listed off my various peccadilloes, punctuated with references from my hours spent scrutinizing the holy grail of fucked-up brains, the *Diagnostic and Statistical Manual of Mental Disorders*.

Dr. Sanders sat for a moment and looked at me, taking in the first bits of information I offered up.

"You know," she said, "I had another client once, and she only ate things that were white. White bread, white potatoes, white corn. Now that's a real eating disorder."

From that comment on, I shut down like a union worker on strike. My mother dragged me to session after session, but instead of talking, I stared over Dr. Sander's head, grunted, and took loud, dramatic breaths whenever she asked me a question. In a last-ditch attempt to get me to say something, she pointed to a feelings poster hanging on her wall, with a series of cartoon faces all scrunched into expressions like "irritated," "furious," "confused," and "ashamed."

"How are you feeling today?" she said, almost begging for a response.

I cocked my head sideways, feigned a good look at the poster, and said, "Where's the face for, 'This is a waste of my fucking time?'"

Dr. Sanders, apparently, agreed. She diagnosed me with an anxiety and depressive disorder and told my mother that she was wasting her money on a psychologist because what I really needed was a psychiatrist. I didn't argue. All I wanted was to be left alone, to be less space.

A few days later, I was in a psychiatrist's office, watching him skim my chart.

"You've been through a lot," he said. "Let's see if we can help you with that." He wrote me a script and told me to call him if I experienced any of the side effects listed on the pamphlet.

The first prescription made me nauseous and I sent myself home from school. Back to the psychiatrist and onto the next drug. That one put me to sleep, so we tried another, but it made my heart pound and my mind race. We stopped that one and tried two more. After a few weeks, I told the doctor my hair was falling out, and he referred me to an endocrinologist. Later, I told him my stomach burned, and he referred me to a gastroenterologist.

By the time school let out, a cocktail of new prescriptions pulsed through my veins.

"How do you feel today?" the psychiatrist asked at a follow-up.

"Fine," I said.

At our check-in, one month later.

"How do you feel today?"

"Fine."

Two months later.

"How do you feel today?"

"Fine."

Six months later.

"How do you feel today?"

"Fine."

"Come back if anything changes."

"Fine."

3

It is February 1. I am thirty years old today. Woot woot. Har har.

Soon, I'll have been alive for twice as long as my father existed in my world. He lived for 5,632 days of my life. On July 3, the anniversary of his death, I will have survived 5,633 days without him.

I pour the last of a bottle of Chablis, his favorite wine, into an empty glass. Every year, I drink a bottle on my birthday, his birthday, and the day he died. He drank Chablis from the box, with those vacuum-sealed metallic bladders stuffed into cardboard. A carton always lived in our fridge, ready and waiting to be trickled into a water glass full of ice. I buy bottles and use stemware, at least, because the job of a daughter is to fix the sins of her father.

Buffy snarls at my foot, insisting on her evening walk despite my wine-soaked plans. I try to ignore her long enough to finish the glass, but her growls turn into aggressive nips, a side effect of her former life as a scrappy Long Island street dog.

"It's a good thing you're cute," I tell her, my tipsy fingers leashing her up.

On the elevator ride down to the street, I prep my best sober voice for my nightly phone call to my mother, a ritual that developed thanks to the convenient time difference between New York and Reno. I dial the number while Buffy beelines to lift her leg on a pile of garbage, stopping mid-stream to lunge at a passing German Shepherd. I pull at her leash and force her across the street from my apartment building, with her barking like all hell behind me.

"I hear the Demon Dog is being her usual self," my mother says.

"This morning, she broke into my closet, pulled out my laundry, and ate the crotch out of all my underwear. Happy birthday to me."

"They say dogs are a mirror of their owner's personality. That dog would be dead if she'd been adopted by anyone except you."

"That makes both of us," I mumble to myself, thinking about the 5.58 second fall from my window.

"What did you say, honey?"

"Nothing."

I go silent on the other end of the phone. My apartment building is now across the street, little squares of light peppering the building's façade. I count six floors down from the roof, three apartments over from the right, and find my window. It seems so small from down here, so unimportant next to all the other squares of light. It's been thirty-five days since I pushed myself halfway out that window, looking to escape the weight of the life lived behind it. Thirty-five days since the icy wind changed my course, boring the question into my brain, *who am I if I'm not on antidepressants?*

"Did you do anything for your birthday?" my mother says, breaking my trance. I cradle the phone between my ear and shoulder and squat down to pick up Buffy's daily contribution to the noxious Manhattan streets.

"Got into another fight about the bakery, so it was a typical day. Yay, business partnership."

"You two have been fighting since the day the place opened."

"If I can just shut up for another year and a half, then I can blame the wreckage on the expiring lease and vow to never have a business partner again," I say, dropping Buffy's poop bag onto an already overflowing garbage can.

"I wish there was something I could do."

"Turn back time," I say.

"I'm so sorry, honey. Maybe tomorrow will be better."

"Unlikely."

"Try and enjoy the rest of your night. I love you."

"You too."

I hang up the phone and head back to my apartment. On our way to the elevator, Buffy stops to say hi to the night doorman, a Bosnian transplant named Srdjo. He lights up at the sight of her and she accepts an ear scratch, temporarily eschewing her Demon Dog personality.

"Leetle Buffy, the best part 'ov my day! And Brookie," I smile at the endearing way Srdjo pronounces my name, "I have pharmacy for you."

Srdjo stops scratching Buffy and rolls his chair to a box that's filled with pharmaceutical deliveries. He plucks my plump bag out of the crowd, hands it to me, and returns to Buffy.

"Have a good night, Miss Buffy. And you too, Brookie."

I cradle the bag of pills under my arm as Buffy and I go into the elevator. I close my eyes when the doors close, imagining the ride zipped into 5.56 seconds, but the elevator lurches up with a crawl.

Who was I before the antidepressants?

I rack my brain for a memory, any memory, of a time before I was medicated. It's blank, mostly, like the lightbulb of my past is on the fritz and I can only root around for memories when the bulb flickers.

I see a flash of myself in the springtime, learning to weed daffodils with my mother, when a bee comes buzzing at me. My mother drops her scissors into a paper bag filled with scraggly roots and kneels next to me, the threat still zooming around us.

"Close your eyes," my mother says. "Imagine a big beam of white light—the whitest, brightest light—and see it shining out from inside you and surrounding your whole body. The bees can see the white light, sweetie. All you have to do is surround yourself and ask the bees not to hurt you."

I lunge into her and wrap my arms around her thighs, knowing my mother just taught me something that matters, and that most everyone else won't ever understand it. There is something different about her world, I know. I squeeze her tight and refuse to let go.

I see a flash of myself on Halloween. I am six, maybe seven. The lights are off when I come up to our house, and all the pumpkins my mother and I carved together are smashed. Candle wax covers the pumpkin pieces strewn across the front steps. My heart drops, the bag of candy suddenly less sweet. I start to cry and point to the pumpkins. She scoops me up and brings me inside.

"Daddy had a tantrum," she says to me. "Your daddy's father never let him go trick-or-treating. And even though your daddy is a grown up now, it still makes him sad."

I see a flash of myself hunched over a burnt-orange rock polisher as my father reaches his callused hands into the treasure pot of shiny, shimmering pebbles. The rocks we gathered from the river, once covered in mucky silt, now glimmer with swirls of blue and green and flecks of pyrite.

"See how smooth they are," my father says to me, holding up an oval pebble. "That's the work of the rock polisher." He clears his throat and points to the tumbler grit inside the barrel. "This shakes the rocks and they grind against the grit and it smooths out their rough edges." Then he reaches his muddy hand down his shorts and scratches himself.

I open my eyes when the elevator reaches the thirtieth floor, but when the doors start to move, they get stuck. The elevator tries again, jiggles itself up and down until it aligns with the hallway, and the doors slide all the way open. My father could probably fix that. His whole world was mechanical and he knew how to fit it together. The inner workings of machines—the gears and circuits all interacting to bring an inanimate object to life—were so much more interesting to him than the outside world. I think about my mind's gears and circuits as I unleash Buffy and step out of the elevator, how the little dopamine and serotonin molecules fit into receptors, how synapses fire and go dormant at will. My brain feels tired and rusty, in need of a good oiling and parts replacement. My father could fix so many things. I wonder, if he was still here, if he could fix me.

Buffy bolts down the hallway, barks at the door until I open it, and sprints to the couch. I follow her with my wine and laptop, relieved to have reached the part of the day when all there is to do is let the edges of my body melt into the cushions. I log on to Facebook and let my eyes glaze over with the mindless dribble of babies and politics and shitty photos of greasy tacos. It all seems so futile, so empty. Nothing more than desperate hearts screaming through screens in vain hope of feeling something like love.

I don't know how long I scroll. I only stop when a Facebook ad for a company called Remote Year pops up in my feed. I gaze at the ad's island landscape and simple text that reads, "12 months. 12 countries. Travel the world while working remotely." I don't think. I don't Google. I simply click "Learn More," let my fingers fly across the keyboard, and hit "submit."

This isn't abnormal. Every time my business partner and I get into a fight I apply to something in order to parachute out of my situation—an eleven-dollar-an-hour job as a kitchen manager at McMurdo Station in Antarctica, a part-time goat sitter at a homestay in the Swiss Alps, a chance to compete on the blockbuster Food Network show *Chopped*. Something about even considering these opportunities feels scornfully delicious, like sneaking a generous sip of a snotty colleague's overpriced scotch while he's flirting with the bartender. It's not like I ever get chosen for these things. If I did, I couldn't actually go. My life is rooted in New York. I am contractually obligated to a lease for a brick-and-mortar business that makes a physical product. I have a business partner, on paper anyway. We have bills to pay. My apartment building does not allow subleases. I have a dog. Even if I could delete all those factors, jobwise I am qualified for nothing. I make cupcakes for a living and bring home a pauper's salary. It isn't ever going to happen, but I want out. Now. So I down the rest of my wine and revel in the fantasy.

4

The problem isn't that I apply to life-altering opportunities with no obvious plan of execution. The problem is this time, I get chosen. Twice.

First, an email from Remote Year appears in my inbox: "Final Round Acceptance—Congratulations!" Then a casting producer from *Chopped* contacts me after receiving my Chablis-induced application. "I'd love to bring you in next week for an on-camera interview. Your bakery background could work well with some of our crazy ingredients on *Chopped*."

For Remote Year, all I need to do to land an interview for one of the coveted, work-around-the-world spots is fork up a $50 application fee and answer a series of essay questions. If the company even exists. I'm not convinced. A quick Google search brings back only fluff marketing pieces. Any mention of the company from actual participants focuses on all the problems, like how the internet in La Paz, Bolivia was shoddy and how everyone got altitude sickness. There are also posts about how a few participants got fired from their jobs within the first couple of months, as well as complaints about clashing personalities and apartments that weren't livable. In short, the whole thing appears to be a clusterfuck.

The *Chopped* email is more official. According to the message, the interview is casual and comfortable—no cooking required. All I have to do is show up to a studio wearing anything other than blue (the interview room is blue) and chat with the casting team about "you, your cooking, and why you love to do what you do. The only thing you can do wrong is not be yourself!"

Just be myself? "Myself" is suicidal and depressed. What riveting television!

I slam my computer shut and fling it into the corner of the couch. It hits a throw pillow and ricochets off the cushion and into the coffee table before landing on the floor with a thud. I want to pick it up and slam it down, again and again until it is nothing more than a pile of shattered circuits. I want to destroy it so it doesn't remind me of all the people I could be if only I wasn't suicidal and depressed. I could be a world traveler. I could be a *Chopped* champion. I could be free of the frosting-coated prison I created for myself. I could be happy—if only I wasn't me.

I order a large pizza, sip on a glass of wine, and settle into *Dateline*. Lester Holt's familiar baritone voice surrounds me, "When a college co-ed is found dead, police are pulled in multiple directions: a boyfriend, a roommate, and a fellow art student. Who killed Shelley?"

It was the roommate, Lester. Stabbed her in a jealous rage.

Another rerun.

I turn off the TV and heave the remote control across the room. It hits the wall and bursts into a shower of plastic and AAA batteries. I look around my apartment, walls scuffed with eight years of living, furniture sunk and faded, windows so dirty from New York City weather and soot that each morning the unwelcome sun begs to fill the room, and fails.

How did I get here? I should be excited to have two potential opportunities. Instead, all I can think about is falling out my window.

I think back to five years ago, when my business partner and I sat across from each other in a dingy Manhattan deli on a miserable, wet day in February. We were debriefing after I spent the entirety of a meeting in tears, overwhelmed with the amount of money, stress, and time needed to turn a bakery from a side project into a reality. Silence hung between us and seemed to illuminate all the things we did not know about business and each other.

"I know you want to do this," she said, "but I'm not sure you want to do this with me."

My body tingled with a perplexing mix of truth and shame. She was right. But I couldn't admit it, to her or myself. I was too young, dumb, and blind. I didn't want to run a business alone and, even more so, I didn't want to hurt my friend. We were friends, once. Fast friends. Back when our differing views on everything from money to time invested to business advisers seemed small and inconsequential given that we didn't have anything to lose. Besides, New

York City wastes no time initiating the wide-eyed, hopeful souls who choose to start a business there. Misery, to some degree, is a guarantee. I figured we may as well be miserable together and, if the whole thing imploded, I could always go back to considering suicide as a career option.

And here I am four years later, 5.58 seconds away from that reality.

I grab my computer off the floor and watch my email flicker back to consciousness. I agree to show up for the *Chopped* interview, even though I'm sure there's no way I'll get chosen. I've been doing the depressed dance long enough to know I can act my way through appropriate social interaction, but *Chopped* contestants are required to use a basket of mystery ingredients to cook savory appetizers and entrées. I've been baking cupcakes—and nothing else—for five years. My technical skills aren't up to snuff.

Still, I feel a sense of obligation. If I'm going to spend my nights applying to kamikaze moonshots that might launch me out of my life, I may as well follow through. If nothing else, having appointments on my calendar keeps me from going out the window tonight.

After sending off the *Chopped* email, I keep the momentum going and charge the $50 Remote Year application fee to my credit card. When Remote Year asks me to describe my work situation, and how my employer will support a year of working remotely across twelve international locations, I bend the truth until it just about snaps. The bakery's basic marketing responsibilities, which primarily include coming up with baking puns and slapping logos on Instagram posts, becomes "overseeing all digital media and graphic design." The ten minutes I spend inputting receipts into our accounting software becomes "managing all finances and day-to-day business operations." Then I list all the glossy magazines we've been featured in and mention that Google is our client. So what if they only ordered from the bakery twice. Four years ago. And only because I was sleeping with a Googler.

Remote Year accepts my application in three days. I interview with a mousy twenty-four-year-old who calls in from Buenos Aires. Rather, I sit quietly for twenty minutes while she explains how Remote Year works. Essentially, it's a glorified travel agency, but instead of a bus full of retirees hopping from one city to another for a ten-day vacation, it's a bus full of working professionals hopping to twelve international locations, one each month for an entire year. For $2,000 a month, Remote Year handles the pain-in-the-ass part of travel (accommodation, flights, a workspace with reliable internet) while also providing a consistent community of like-minded people. It's a steal, she says, given that $2,000 can't get you a decent one-bedroom apartment in most major American cities.

"Do you have any questions?" she says, prompting me to speak for the first time. I still don't see a world in which I can make this fantastical trip work, but I bring up the bad press about the poor living conditions in La Paz out of curiosity.

"We took La Paz off the itinerary," she says.

"Fair enough," I say, figuring the next time I hear from her, it'll be in the form of a rejection letter.

But two weeks later she emails me to say I've been accepted into a program kicking off in Kuala Lumpur, Malaysia on September 1. From there we will head to Thailand, Cambodia, Croatia, Czech Republic, Portugal, Mexico, Colombia, Peru, and finally Argentina. Ten countries. Twelve cities. One year. The group will be named "Libertatum," she says, the Latin word for "freedom."

When I finish reading her email, I walk to my window and open it. The screen still rests against the wall, hidden behind an anthurium rustling in the breeze. I stick my torso out the window and watch traffic move like lava inching toward open water. People mill about thirty floors below, creating the same patterns in the sidewalk they did yesterday and the day before and the day before. From up here in the faded afternoon sun, it's almost as if this world is orderly.

I like orderly. I like knowing that every morning, coffee steeps in my French press while I walk Buffy around the block. I like knowing that every day we stop to say hi to Richard, a homeless man who sits in his wheelchair, jostling a few coins in his beat-up Dunkin' Donuts cup on the corner of 38th and 3rd. Someone from the shelter drops him off after sunrise and picks him up every evening. He doesn't have a cardboard sign asking for a miracle or a little compassion or $35 for the bus fare home. He's simply an old man watching the world change.

"I've been on this corner thirty years!" he often tells me, swelling with pride. Some days I buy him coffee. Other days he hands me a few coins and asks me to buy a cup for him. He scratches Buffy's chin with his long, yellow fingernails. But lately he's been showing up on the corner with an oxygen tank and tubes running into his nose. His eyes are misty with cataracts, two clouds floating over a dark night. His beard has turned white. His voice is thinning and I wonder if a year from now Richard will still be here. If I will still be here.

I like knowing that when Buffy and I return home, my coffee is ready. I like taking a sip to erase the taste of gel capsules on my tongue. My medications are timed down to the hour and missing a window of time is like injecting a week's worth of coffee directly into my veins. Would I even be able to get the right drugs on a remote island in Thailand or a sleepy Argentinian town?

From up on the thirtieth floor, looking down, with the February cold prickling at my face, a thought rides in on the tail of the wind: *I never actually made the choice to go on these drugs in the first place. I was a child. Fifteen years old. Grieving my father's death. I just did what the adults told me to do.*

Suddenly a flood of questions comes at me.

Why am I still on the same drugs I was on when I was a teenager? I don't wear the same clothes as when I was fifteen, so why am I still on the same medications? Shouldn't they have changed as my brain changed? What were the doctors thinking? What was I thinking? How might my life be different? How might I be different? Is this who I really am? Or is this just who I have come to believe I am? What drugs do I actually need to be on? Do I even need them at all? Who am I if I'm not on brain-altering medication?

In one crystalizing moment I realize I am left with only two choices: keep taking the drugs and stay on this path, which, if nothing changes, leads toward suicide; or get off the drugs and leave my business partner, my dog, and the person I thought I knew. I pull my body back into my apartment and try to put the screen in place, but the wood is twisted and the sliding mechanism is stuck so I kick the screen against the wall and scream "fuck!" when it scuffs the paint.

Then I run to my computer and put the $5,000 down payment for Remote Year on my credit card. The charge clears. Everything and nothing has changed.

5

I am on the corner of Lexington and 41st Street, standing in front of gold revolving doors with ornate metal swirls that hold the fears and thoughts of the tens of thousands of people who pass through its turnstile, day after day. I have been here before. Thousands of times. This is my favorite entrance to Grand Central Station, hidden in the foundation of a sky rise, known only to New Yorkers who know where to look.

I enter here because this building holds slivers of everything I am. The pharmacy in the basement has seen me late into the night, searching the aisles for Plan B and nail polish. The realtors who stumbled upon the empty space that would one day become the bakery are on the twentieth floor. The focus groups that exchanged forty dollars for my opinion on cell phones or dog food all met here, too. Today I am here to meet my new psychiatrist, Dr. Chin. Though I've been in this building many times before, when I fill out the doormen's security form asking me who I am, what I want, and where I'm going, I feel embarrassed to scribble down that I am going to a psychiatrist. As I slide the clipboard back to the guards, I wonder, *Are they curious about what is wrong with me? Do they think of me at all?*

Security gives me a name tag, leads me to the elevator embossed with gold and silver art-deco geese, and sends me to my floor. The elevator takes me up to a large waiting room with plastic armchairs, one receptionist, and a single plant begging for water.

"Hello, my name is . . . " I say to the receptionist, but she hands me a clipboard before I can finish. I fill out my forms, and the receptionist tells me my doctor will be with me shortly.

A woman dressed in a dull, gray pantsuit appears, her black hair pulled back into a lifeless knot. She calls my name without looking up from her chart. I stand and her black eyes rise just as I get near enough to say, "Hello, my name is . . . ," and she turns away and I follow her until we arrive in her small, square, drab office. There is a couch and a bookshelf, and certificates hang on the wall. She sits in a chair in front of her desk, cross-legged, a clog hanging off one foot.

"I'm Dr. Chin. Are we billing this to insurance or are you paying out of pocket?" she asks.

"Insurance," I say.

"Insurance card?"

I dig through my wallet for my card and hand it to her.

"Your copay is $50. How will you be paying?"

"Credit card."

She holds out her hand for my credit card, runs it, and hands me the receipt to sign. Through all of this, she's hardly seen my face.

"Okay, so what are you here for?"

"The short of it is I've been on antidepressants for about fifteen years. My father died suddenly when I was a teenager, and I was put on the drugs a few months later."

Dr. Chin makes a note on my chart, but says nothing, so I keep talking to fill the silence.

"I have an opportunity to travel around the world for a year. I don't know if I can even pull it off, but if I do, I figure I can't take a suitcase full of prescriptions across borders. I'm here to see what my options are. Maybe see what I'm like without them."

"As long as you have a prescription from me," she says, "you should be able to get the medications anywhere."

"Even on a remote island in Thailand?"

Dr. Chin lifts her eyes without moving her head and stares at me. "Why do you want to get off them anyway?"

"I've been on them for half my life, for my entire adult life. I want to know if they're even doing anything because honestly I'm still fucking depressed."

"Perhaps the prescription needs to be tweaked," Dr. Chin says as she scribbles something and moves onto her next question. "Have you ever had suicidal thoughts?"

I know my way around this question, and I know I have to be careful. Admitting any sort of plan sometimes triggers a doctor or therapist to place an involuntary, seventy-two-hour hold on a patient deemed at risk for suicide. I can tell her yes, I've experienced occasional suicidal thoughts, but I cannot tell her I stand at my thirty-story window and watch for breaks in sidewalk traffic that leave the cement wide open. I cannot tell her I hide my assortment of chef's knives in the back of my cupboard because I hone the blade to cut through sinewy flesh. I cannot tell her that while beef needs to be slit side to side, against the muscle grain, a wrist needs long, parallel strokes.

I look her in the eye and lie. "I don't have a plan, if that's what you're asking."

It's enough to get Dr. Chin to move on.

"Have you ever thought about hurting someone else?"

"Well, I'm a New Yorker, so I regularly think about punching people in the face."

She stares at me, unamused. "I generally don't recommend people stop taking their medication, especially under this amount of stress and change."

"Tough shit for me then." I am already annoyed with this woman and her glib, box-checking attitude. "Something about what's going on with me isn't working. I don't know if it's the wrong antidepressants or if these ones don't work anymore or if I'm just so fucked in the head that this is how it's going to be, forever. I don't see how I'm supposed to get the answer to any of those questions without getting off the prescriptions to figure out my baseline. I've tried to get off them before, without seeing a psychiatrist, but . . . "

Dr. Chin stops me. "Why didn't you do it under the care of a psychiatrist?"

"My general practitioner has been prescribing to me for seven years. When I tried to taper off them a few years ago, he told me to cut the Wellbutrin in half and . . . "

"You can't cut Wellbutrin in half," she interrupts. "The version you're on is time-released, so when you cut it in half, you break the chemical chain and mess with that release. To taper off you'd have to take a smaller dose."

"He didn't tell me that."

"If you decide to move forward with this, I think it would be better for you to try going off them one by one, starting with the Effexor because you're already on the lowest dose so we can't taper. The Effexor is more likely than the Wellbutrin to have withdrawal effects."

"What kind of effects?"

"I've heard it's a little like having the flu. Occasionally people report a sort of electric shock in the brain."

I let out a quiet laugh of perplexing self-pity and think back to the last time I accidentally skipped a dose. It was nothing like the flu. I was out of refills and it was Saturday. My doctor's office was closed. Within a few hours of missing my usual dose my heart seemed to twitch right out of my chest. I snapped at a waitress and broke out into cold sweats. Then I ran to the pharmacy and begged for a few days of pills to get me through until I could call my doctor on Monday. Following the conversation with the pharmacist was like hearing someone speak underwater. But he gave me the drugs. I washed them down dry, in the drugstore, right next to a display of laxatives.

As my heart slowed and my body equalized and the familiar desensitized hum washed over me, I thought, *I need these pills. Without them, my heart explodes and my mind shuts down. Without them, I'm soaked with rage and filth. Without them, I am nothing but who I am.*

Now, in Dr. Chin's office, I wonder if it was just the early stages of antidepressant withdrawal.

"How long does all of this last?" I ask her.

She shrugs. "I can't really say. A few days. Maybe a week. It's different from person to person, but I can prescribe you Prozac to help manage those side effects."

"Prozac? I don't understand how the solution to getting off psychiatric drugs is more psychiatric drugs."

"Effexor XR has an extremely short half-life, which means it doesn't stay in the body very long. A small number of people experience intense withdrawal, but because the medication leaves the system after a day or so, it shouldn't last long. The other meds stay in your body for a while, so you may not feel the effects of not having them in your system for a few weeks."

"Then wouldn't it be better to suck it up and deal with the side effects if it's only going to last a few days rather than take another brain-altering medication I've never been on and will have to get off as well?"

Dr. Chin shrugs. "You could if you wanted to, I guess. I'll write you a prescription for Prozac, regardless. Stop taking the Effexor and see how it goes. If the withdrawal symptoms are bad, take the Prozac. Here's my card. Call the office if you have questions and let's make an appointment for a month from now."

I take the card and the script for Prozac, my stomach turning at the thought of adding yet another drug to my repertoire. We make an appointment for one month from today and I put the time and date in my calendar and ask her to call or email me with an appointment reminder.

"I don't do appointment reminders," she says without elaborating.

I figure the receptionist will handle it. "Um, okay. See you in a month, I guess?"

I gather my things and Dr. Chin mutters "good luck" on my way out.

In the waiting room, the plant is screaming for water. I ask the receptionist if she can send me an appointment reminder, but she shakes her head without looking at me and says, "Nah. I don't do that. Maybe your doctor will though."

I point to the plant behind me and say, "That plant. It needs water. Please have someone give it some."

She cocks her head and twists her body to look past me, to the plant standing helpless on the other side of the room. "I don't know who's in charge of that, but it's not me."

"But it needs water."

"I'll tell the janitor."

I sigh and head for the elevator. The plant won't be there in a month. It will shrivel and brown and turn from plump to brittle until someone finally notices it and throws it into the dumpster. I want to steal it away from the fluorescent lighting and take it the few blocks back to my apartment and place it in the morning sun, watering it gently at first so as not to flood its parched roots. Watering it slowly until it understands it is safe and it can drink as much as it needs. Watering it until it knows the water will always come, and each morning the sun will rise on its leaves, until after a lifetime lived under artificial light, it will finally have the chance to bloom.

～～～～～～～～

I chicken out the next morning and swallow my Effexor along with all the rest. I have a little more than five months before I board a plane to Malaysia. What's one more day? Besides, I need all my mental facilities to get through my on-camera *Chopped* interview. With the non-refundable, $5000 Remote Year deposit burning in the back of my mind, I can't dismiss the potential of a $10,000 prize courtesy of Food Network, even if getting chosen is a long shot.

I put on my best not-blue jacket and take Buffy to the twenty-sixth floor of my apartment building before heading to the casting studio. We come here every day. Buffy knows exactly where she is and darts down the hallway to 26F, her little tail wagging with such force her rump seems ready to take off like a helicopter.

I ring the doorbell, and a faint "coming!" chimes from deep within the apartment. On the other side of the door I hear shuffling and the rattle of a chain lock. Buffy jumps at the door, scratching at the knob as it turns.

"Ohhhh, Buffy!" Dolores squeals as the dog uses her snout to push the door open and let herself in. Dolores is a pudgy, arthritic widow with wild, gray hair who refuses to trade her independence for the ease of assisted living. She moves with a cane, yet Buffy never gets caught under her feet. The two have been spending their days together for almost five years, ever since the bakery opened and my workdays stretched to fourteen hours. At first, I left Buffy alone in our apartment, but she barked all day and pissed off the neighbors. I tried doggy day care, but she was kicked out for picking fights with other dogs. Knowing the majority of tenants in my apartment complex were living out their golden years, I slipped a note under each of the 264 units asking if anyone spent most of their day at home and would like a little canine companionship.

Dolores responded, "I would love to meet your sweet little pup! Come say hi. 26F."

Five years later, both Buffy and Dolores get cranky if they don't see each other every day. Dolores' slow pace and serene demeanor soothes Buffy's surly personality, and she transforms into a different dog in the presence of the old woman.

"You're looking stylish today," Dolores says to me. Buffy is standing behind her, ears perked and tail wagging.

"Thank you," I give Dolores a little twirl. "I have an interview downtown. I'll be back in a few hours. Is that okay?"

"Oh yes, we're just fine. I made hot dogs. Buffy likes hot dogs."

"Just a little. She's looking rather porky lately."

"She's just stout, is all," Dolores says, waving goodbye. She closes the door and I hear the two of them shuffle off into her apartment.

As I make my way downtown, it occurs to me that I cannot take Buffy and Dolores away from each other. Buffy's proclivity for biting people's feet makes her impossible to re-home, and I won't surrender her to a shelter. Dolores, meanwhile, has flourished in the years she and Buffy have spent together. She started swimming every morning and got herself on the internet. She sends regular group emails to her friends and family with pictures and updates about Buffy. Their bond is stronger than my desire to blow up my life and flee the country. I'll eat the $5,000 Remote Year deposit before I separate them. Still, full time canine care is a lot to ask from an eighty-six-year-old woman. I decide I'll broach the topic with Dolores's daughter, Sarah, after the *Chopped* interview. Maybe together we can find a solution.

At the casting studio, a producer, Maya, brings me into a small room with a large camera and sits me down on a tall stool. We cover the basics: name and age, place of employment, length of time in the culinary world. Even though I've seen the show, she also runs through the format: four chefs compete against each other in a three-round contest. At the beginning of each round (appetizer, entrée, and dessert), the chefs are given a mystery basket filled with unusual ingredients like fish collars, peach pits, leftover Kung Pao chicken, and the tears of virgins—all of which must be featured in the dish. At the end of the time limit (twenty minutes for the appetizer, thirty for the entrée and dessert), the chefs' dishes are evaluated by a panel of judges who ultimately decide which plate ends up on the chopping block. The chef who made the chopped dish goes home early and empty handed. The last chef standing wins.

"What would you do with the money?" Maya asks. She's about the same age as me, with dark hair, big eyes, and an energy that is both friendly and straightforward.

"I actually just got an opportunity to travel around the world for a year," I say.

"I bet $10,000 would help with that."

"It would. We bakers aren't known for our riches. I'm supposed to leave in five months. Not sure if that would be an issue for filming."

"I'll make a note about when you're supposed to leave," Maya says. "Now, tell me about the most creative dish you cooked recently."

I don't answer right away. It's been years since I cooked with any joy or creativity. At the bakery, I am a robot of my own creation, baking and frosting thousands of identical cupcakes, day after day. By the time I get home, my definition of cooking is ordering takeout. I decide there's no point in lying to her. The last thing I want to do is embarrass myself on national TV, so she may as well know I'm out of cooking shape.

"Honestly, I don't think I've turned my stove on since the day the bakery opened. But I once transformed the humble bacon, lettuce, and tomato sandwich into a cold summer soup made with romaine lettuce purée, confit tomatoes, pork belly lardons, and breadcrumbs fried in bacon fat. People liked it. It was in another life, though. I'm sure there are plenty of actual chefs more qualified to compete, given I don't cook much anymore."

"Food Network ultimately decides who gets chosen, and they're always looking for women, since there's so few in the industry. You might have a shot."

"That's terrifying," I say.

"Makes for great television, though."

"So this is entertainment first and cooking second?"

Maya smirks. "If you've already figured that out, you're ahead of the rest. Don't overthink it."

"I can always say no if I decide it's too much, right?"

"Of course. If I were you, I'd forget about it and get your life in order for that trip. We'll reach back out if they want you and the timing works out."

I take Maya's advice and put *Chopped* out of my head, an easy task given more pressing issues like tapering off the antidepressants and talking to Dolores about taking Buffy. As soon as I leave the interview, I call Sarah, who I've come to know over the years during her visits to Dolores. I tell her about Remote

Year, about how I don't want to take Buffy and Dolores away from each other but don't know how the logistics would work.

"Don't worry about it," Sarah says without hesitation. "We'll figure it out. Mom and Buffy are going to be just fine. You go have an amazing experience."

I feel the color drain from my face. Sarah's blessing shifts Remote Year from abstract to concrete, the realization of what's about to happen finally hitting me. I say goodbye to Sarah and open an app on my phone. Against a yellow-and-pink, confetti background, the number 447: the number of days until my bakery's lease is up. Underneath the number, in serif font: FREEDOM! I swipe to another screen, to a big number gently laid over a photo of a wave just seconds from tickling the arm of a bright-red starfish sunbathing in sand: 19,600 days until I die. I open a new countdown and plug in Remote Year's start date—September 1. I have 176 days to change the course of my entire life.

Staring at this number, it's like I separate from my body, the weight of change too much for me to process. I watch a ghost of myself get on the subway and head back to my building. I see myself go into my apartment and sit, the sound of street noise echoing from down below. Time loses all meaning, and I jolt awake a few hours later, my apartment dark, body still disconnected from my mind.

Bleary eyed, I watch myself go to Dolores's apartment and settle into her living room, Buffy squeaking a plush duck toy on the floor.

"I have some news," I hear myself say. "I got an opportunity to travel around the world for a year. Starting in Malaysia. Ending in Argentina. I'd be leaving at the end of the summer."

"How exciting," Dolores says, a worried smile appearing on her wrinkled face. She shifts on the couch, looks at Buffy. "But what will happen to Buffy?"

"She'll stay here, with you, where she belongs. If that's what you want, of course. I already talked to Sarah. We'll make sure she has a consistent walker, if you're not always up for it."

Dolores sighs with relief, the smile brightening. "Oh good! We're quite the pair, she and I. We nap a lot."

"I know. It's like she's been yours all along, and I'm just a glorified dog walker."

"We're going to have so much fun!" Dolores squeals, clapping her hands. Buffy releases the stuffed duck from her toothy grasp and smacks her lips. She looks at me. Looks at Dolores. Then walks over to Dolores's feet and sits.

"I think that's her way of telling us she's okay with this decision," I say, relief and heartbreak bringing me back into my body.

"She is an expressive little pup," Dolores says, her chest puffing with pride.

I think about the antidepressants in my bathroom four floors above, waiting patiently for each new morning when they are called to duty.

"I guess I have to do this now," I say.

Dolores smiles, scratches Buffy's ears, and says, "That's what youth is for."

6

I look to the clouds and watch as the sky drips.

Drip, drip, drip.

It is evening. I have been without Effexor XR for four days. The first day is unremarkable. The second day I shake. The third day is hot and cold and hot and cold. Today I am only hot. My arms are bare for the first time this year. I am walking to my apartment when the rain comes, without warning.

Drip, drip, drip.

All around me, the whoosh and click of umbrellas opening in dramatic, staccato beats. My umbrella is at home. The rain hurts my skin.

This is new.

My eye catches an aluminum lamppost hovering over Park Avenue like a cobra ready to strike. Light glows through like it always does but now I see something different: the lightbulb. This is the first time in eight years I've noticed the lightbulb. Bulbous edges and tiny coils peek out from its root.

Drip, drip, drip.

In one breath something shifts. A fog lifts. My senses turn razor-sharp. Headlights refract in piercing, angular starbursts so bright I have to squint. A siren wails and my ears pound. The metallic taste of bile gathers in the back of my throat. Exhaust prickles my nose. Individual raindrops. A million little bullets. Edges.

Each droplet stings.

It has been six days since I stopped taking Effexor XR and there is bloodshed in the street. I am on 38th Street and it is daylight and there is blood, so much blood, running down the sidewalks in ruby tendrils twinkling in the sun's light. The blood belongs to a man I don't know. A man who just a few moments before was on his way to his job, his lunch, his family, but who now lies crumpled before my feet thanks to the knife in my hand that slit him from ear to ear. A pool of blood wells up around my shoes and seeps in between my toes, sticky warm life escaping from its host. People pass all around us, white wires dangling from their ears, shoulders hunched, head down to the ground and eyes on their screen. They don't notice me and they don't notice the man and they instinctively go left or right to avoid us in a rehearsed, unspoken dance only New Yorkers know.

I step over the man and leave him to bleed.

I take a breath and walk a few more steps toward Lexington Avenue when I'm stalled by an elderly woman pushing a walker. She is slow and unaware. I find a break in the crowd coming toward us and, passing her, I kick her walker out from underneath her and she topples and crashes headfirst into a metal fence protecting a Callery pear tree from pissing dogs. The coiled edge of the fence lodges into her temple and her blood drains into the earth, but the wheels on her walker keep spinning and the sound of them grates so I grab the walker and raise it over my head and slam it down on the old woman. The walker snaps and her bones break and the soil swells, saturated with blood, but no one on the street looks up.

This must be the real you. This is who you are without medication. You want to take lives. And this will never, ever go away. Get back to the drugs. Get back to what you know.

There is a baby in a stroller. I rip it out of its harness and swing it by the ankles into a parked car. Its mother just nods at me and pushes the empty stroller along the cracked sidewalk until the wheels hit the old lady's pool of blood and send a stream of red across the mother's face. She turns back to me and smiles.

I pass a small dog tied to a bike rack. The dog looks at me with its black-and-white face cocked sideways, ears perked. I knock it over with my foot and use my bare, bloodied heel to suffocate the creature until it is nothing but a pile of lifeless fur. When I am done with the dog, I take the knife to my own throat and twist it in deep but I am not dead. I go back to the old lady and beat my head into the fence and I am not dead. I run into traffic and finally I am dead and the man and the old woman and the baby and the dog are all with me and we are together but no one notices we are dead because it's all in my head and I can't stop the images from flashing flashing flashing.

The black-and-white dog barks and I am back into the world. The sound of jackhammers, car horns, and building construction suddenly surrounds me like an orchestra from hell and my stomach turns and I can't feel my arms and wherever I am going I can't go there anymore. I turn around and run back toward my apartment. *Make it stop.* Past the drooling dog, the crying baby, the old lady, and the smiling man and back to the safety of my home. *Turn it down.* No one can know. *Turn it off.* It's been a week since I stopped taking the first antidepressant and now this is what I see when I go outside. *They'll put me back on the drugs. They'll lock me up. They'll keep me here. They can't know.*

The elevator is taking too long and I'm shaking and sweating and crying. I fumble for my keys, open the door, slam it shut. I fall into my bed and wail into the pillows, hoping they muffle my cries because my howls are so deep and primal that even in my rage I am shocked at the sound bellowing out of me. I wonder if my white bedspread is absorbent enough to soak up all the blood from the street, but soon the bloodshed gives way to puddles of snot and tears and spit. I rip off my shirt because it is suddenly made of chains and, as I look at the folds in my stomach heaving with each shallow sob, my flesh disgusts me. I want to cut off my hapless breasts and shave off my hips and dig the moles out of my skin until I am whittled down into a thin, straight, smooth line.

I look from the window to the dresser to the closet. Everything I own takes up too much space. The dresser with its half-open drawers is too much space. The hangers, all askew, are too much space. The closet stuffed with old unworn clothes, too much space. I want to stuff the clothes into bags and push the dresser out the door and rid my space of the too much space because it's taking up all of my space.

Everything I create is too much space. The dirt I drag in from outside and the strands of brown hair against the white tile and the splashes of water from the sink and the waste from what I ate and drank. The dust in the corners and the used coffee grounds scattered across the counter and the plastic takeout container wrapped in plastic wrap delivered in a plastic bag with plastic forks thrown into a plastic bin with a plastic liner. It's all too much space.

My breath is too much space. My thoughts are too much space. I am too much space.

I am also nauseous and need to turn over. Hands push down on the bed to create just enough room for me to drag my forehead across the sheets and stop for a rest halfway through, knees tucked into my chest, forearms furled against my throat, shins and cheek pressed into the mattress. The torn remnants of my shirt rest on the wood floor like fallen tombstones. My back is exposed and I am cold, but the sun pours through my window and warms my skin.

Be less space.

I contract my toes and pull my arms in tighter because the warmth of the sun reminds me I am still here and I am alive, but I don't want to be here and right now living hurts so I rock to distract myself from the sun. Outside, an ambulance gets stuck in traffic and, even though I am thirty floors up, the sound ricochets off the buildings and it is so loud it may as well be in the room with me. Louder now and piercing and it's not stopping, but the traffic isn't moving and with each ring my heart pumps faster and I rock harder and this goes on for minutes that feel like hours until the traffic breaks and the sirens escape and I scream "Shut the fuck up!" but the words melt into the noise, unheard.

Be less space.

I close my eyes and am in a desert. All around me is nothing but sand and pebbles and the occasional shrub. I have not been here before but my people were once here. We were walking together for hundreds of miles over hundreds of days, moving from one place to another, all of us. But I fell behind and they left me. I know they are not coming back. They left me because I couldn't keep up. Because I am weak. Because I take up their space. I drop to my knees in the sand and look around for traces of *them*, their leftovers, like the mummified figures in Pompeii. Their footprints have long been taken by the wind.

I will die here.

My jaw is tight and needs to be loosened so I open my mouth as wide as I can and wider still and now my face is twisted and I scream but do not make a sound.

Be less space.

I am starving and empty so my hands grip the earth and I shovel sand into my mouth. The weight piles up in my stomach and my mouth opens wider and my body tries to purge, but the earth is too heavy so I heave and still, I keep shoveling it in until I choke and the wind picks up and the sun beats down and there is no water, there is no water, there is no God.

Be less space. No one can help you. *Be less space.* You're powerless. *Be less space.* You're trapped. *Be less space.* They left you. *Be less space.* They left you to die. *Be less space.* They don't love you enough to come back for you.

Be less space. Be less space. Be less space.

~~~~~~~~~~

I wake up in a ball in the middle of the bed, head where my feet should be. I am large and encumbering. Larger than the bed. Heavier than the building. Pinned to the bedsheets by the force of my mind. Hours pass. Buffy jumps onto the bed and paws my arm. But I don't move. Can't move. So she turns a few circles, curls herself up next to me, and waits. More than anyone or anything else, this little dog has kept me here in this city, here in this body, here on this Earth. But even she has become the target of my murderous thoughts and I can't look at her without seeing her dead at my hand. I close my eyes and feel her, her soft, little body trusting me to be here, to take care of her.

She senses something changing, that I am not quite right. She stays near. Picks fights on the street when people come too close. Whimpers when I leave. Cowers when I sob. When I quiet down, she tucks herself into me and gently licks my hand, toe, chin. I think she would scoop me up and rock me to sleep if she could, like I did when I first brought her home from the shelter, her little lungs stuffed full of pneumonia the rescue agency didn't know she had. We sat together for days, soothing music filling the apartment, Buffy wrapped in a blanket and held warm against my chest. Her already small body seemed to lighten by the minute over the first forty-eight hours, but soon she stabilized enough for me to run to the grocery store and buy a rotisserie chicken. I picked at it while she rested against me, occasionally dangling a morsel near her cocoon of blankets. Finally a snout emerged, sniffing for chicken. Hope.

That same snout nudges me now, her wet nose ice against my cheek. My heart breaks when I think about how I must be hurting her, and I tear up again as I leash her to go out. On the elevator ride to the service entrance, I wonder how many people are out tonight. How many will die in my mind. We walk past a man muttering to himself on the corner and right away I drop Buffy's leash and my hands are around his throat and my thumbs press into the folds of his saggy, freeloading neck and his yellow eyes bulge and his fifth of vodka falls to the ground as he twitches without breath.

The sound of shattering glass startles me back to the night. Buffy's leash is still wrapped around my wrist. She's waiting for me to pick a direction. The man sways side to side with drunken delight, the broken bottle at his feet.

He drops his pants and squats over a bucket.

"The fuck you lookin' at?" he slurs in my general direction. "You wanna watch the show, sweetheart?"

Buffy launches forward to nip at his tattered shoes, but the leash stops her and she chokes. The man breaks into a toothless, full-body laugh, the bucket teetering under his weight. I wonder how much space lies between a man and his bucket and the woman whose mind's eye has a hand around his throat.

We turn away and speed-walk in the opposite direction until we're around the corner, alone. Buffy finds a tree and I call my mother.

"Hi, sweetie," she says. "How are you?"

Words betray me and I sob into the phone, thinking about the guilt my mother would feel if I snapped. I'd be arrested before I could kill myself. I'd end up in prison, plead insanity, and ruin her life. Maybe I'd end up on *Dateline* myself, in an episode titled "Prescription for Murder."

"I can't do this anymore," I heave out, squatting over Buffy's warm pile of shit as tears fall to the cement. "I *need* the drugs. You don't understand. What's going through my mind . . . I . . . I . . . " My breath squeezes into shallow pants, mucous and stomach acid gathering in my throat, pinching my syllables into squeaks. "I don't know how to do this. This was a mistake and if this is who I am without medication, then I can't do it. I can't. I can't be this person. I don't know what she might do."

My mother doesn't pause, doesn't waver.

"Call Kathy. Now. Hang up and I'll text you her number," my mother says. "I love you."

The line goes dead and my phone beeps with Kathy's contact info. Kathy is a psychologist and one of my mother's closest friends. I haven't talked to her in years, but I know I need help. Professional help. I can't call Dr. Chin. It's midnight and all I have is her office number. Besides, if I tell her about my homicidal thoughts, I'm worried she'll put me on an involuntary psychiatric hold.

Buffy waits for my lead while I steady my shaking hands and tie her blue bag of crap into a knot before dropping it into a trashcan on the corner. I pull my hood over my head and turn my face away from the homeless man as we make our way back to my building. Srdjo is on duty. He gives me a gentle nod and soft smile. He tells me if there's anything I need, I shouldn't hesitate to ask. I know he's seen my bloodshot, puffy eyes and I wonder if he's heard the cries from my apartment. I don't ask, and neither does he.

When we get home, Buffy jumps on the couch, flops on her back, and rubs herself against the velveteen cushions. I make my way to the table and dial Kathy's number. Just as she picks up the phone, Buffy hops off the couch and sits at my feet.

"Hi, sweetheart." Kathy's voice is warm honey in a pot of bitter tea. I remember afternoons in her house as a young girl, trying to ride one of her four massive, purebred boxers like a horse. This small, joyful memory sparks through the pain, but burns away as swiftly as it comes.

"Your mom told me you're having a tough time," she says.

"Yeah." Tears come again. "I don't know what she's told you."

"Not much. Just that you saw a psychiatrist and are getting off the antidepressants. What's going on?"

"I'm seeing things in my head." I struggle to get the words out. For a moment I think about not telling her the full truth, but I'm exhausted. I know the only way she might be able to help me is if she knows everything, so I continue. "I'm thinking about hurting people. Really hurting them. Physically. Even my dog. I look at her and I see myself hurting her." Rivers of snot run down my face and pool in the space between my chest and shirt. "It's detailed. Graphic. It won't stop. It happens every time I go outside or see another person. It's all I can think about. What if it stops being in my head? I'm afraid I might actually hurt . . . what if I'm going crazy?"

My words trail off as I think about how everyone in my life would react if I hurt someone. Would they be surprised? Would they say things like, "She never seemed like someone capable of this"? Or would they say, "She always had her demons"? Or maybe they would pass the blame. "If only she had stayed on the meds."

Kathy breaks through my loop of thoughts.

"Honey, it's okay. You're not crazy. You're not going to hurt anyone."

"But how do you know?" I demand.

"The fact that you're so upset and scared of hurting someone means you're not going to hurt anyone. You're aware of what you're thinking. Crazy people don't know they're crazy. What the hell did that doctor say to you?"

"She said because of the type of medication and the dose I was taking, I could only go cold turkey."

"What medication is it?"

"Effexor XR. I'm still on the rest of them."

"Well, she's a fucking idiot."

I'm not entirely sure if Kathy is really not worried about me hurting anyone, or if she's just doing a damn good job of pretending everything is fine. Either way, her voice calms me and my breathing begins to slow. The anxiety around my thoughts gives way to frustration toward Dr. Chin.

"I mean, she offered to prescribe me Prozac while I detoxed, but I wasn't comfortable adding a new drug to my system. Maybe that was stupid, but . . . "

"That was what they put your dad on, right?"

"Yes."

"And he hated it?"

"He said it killed his mind."

"Which is why you didn't want to take it?"

"He had such a bad reaction to it," I say. "If any of this is genetic then maybe it wouldn't have been a good idea, but what if this isn't withdrawal at all. Maybe this is just me. Maybe it is all genetic. Maybe this is who I really am."

Kathy sighs. "I wish you had called me after you talked to Dr. Chin."

"Too late now. It's been over a week. And it's not getting better. It's getting worse."

"It takes time. You can reinstate the Effexor if the withdrawal symptoms are unbearable." I think about taking a pill, but something primal kicks in at the suggestion of swallowing another one of those fuckers.

"As long as this is temporary," I say, my words spoken clear for the first time all night. "I board a plane to Malaysia in 168 days."

"Your mother told me about Remote Year. It sounds like such an adventure!"

"Fuck the adventure. The adventure doesn't matter if I can't get these drugs out of my body and get this over with as fast as I can. Any idea how long this might last?"

"We both know better than to put a timeline on it," she says. "It's just part of getting the meds out of your system. You've been taking some powerful stuff for a long, long time. This is a hard thing you're doing."

I wipe the snot from my nose and sniffle into the phone. "If you talk to my mom, please don't give her any details. I know this is hard for her and I don't want her to think any of it is her fault because it's not her fault and she's already been through so much and she's always there for me, but it's not fair to her and I love her so much and I'm hurting her and . . . "

I trail off and break down again.

"Honey, I promise. I promise I won't tell your mother. And you can call me anytime."

I calm myself long enough to thank Kathy and hang up.

I want to be home. I don't know where home is, but I want to be there, not here. Here is a place filled with uncertainty and I want to be where things are certain because certainty is the backbone of home. Certainty is waking up in a house in the woods to the sound of my father clomping down the stairs with such strength if you hadn't heard it hundreds of times, you were sure the stairs might break under his force. It's walking up from my cold bedroom and into the warmth of the living room, heated by an iron fireplace that has been burning for hours, just like it has every morning. It's letting my childhood dog outside to run and knowing that, despite the cars on the road and bears in the forest, she will always come back as soon as I open the front door and yell for her as loud as I can into the trees, until her little paws come sprinting down the street and up the driveway.

I think about that yelling now, with Buffy scratching her ear at my feet. In calling my childhood dog back from wherever she was, I got to scream as loud as I could and release whatever might have been pent up inside me, into the safety of an untouched forest. But here in Manhattan, I swallow the roaches and rats and shit and piss and noise and anger and stress and greed. I swallow the buildings that once rose as monuments of potential and now sit as gravestones of the past. The business born and strangled on 9 Clinton Street in the Lower East Side. A friendship nurtured in a brownstone in Brooklyn and demolished on a bench in Central Park. A relationship that began here. Another that ended there.

It all teeters on the edge, kept in check by a row of orange bottles guaranteeing just enough. Just enough to go to work. Just enough to smile and wave. Just enough to get wet without noticing the rain. But what happens when the stairs no longer creak and the fire turns to smoke and the dog doesn't return and everything that once held it all together disintegrates into ash that clogs my veins and weighs down my limbs and there's nothing left to do but crumble under its weight?

That weight, at least, was steady. Trapped inside me it was safe.

But now it burns the bottom of my throat, begging to be released.

<hr />

Four weeks without Effexor.

Hunched over the stainless-steel prep table at my bakery, the spot between my right shoulder blade and vertebrae throbs with a familiar burning heat. It's as if someone took a railroad spike and roasted it over an open flame until it was molten orange and then rammed it in between my seventh and eighth rib, an inch or so from my thoracic spine. I crouch against the prep table like a bear scratching itself on a tree and bend my spine into the edge of the table until my back cracks with the pop of a crisp carrot. But my skin is still tender, so I attach ice packs to my back by wrapping my torso in industrial, food-grade cling wrap. When that doesn't work, I sit in the low-boy freezer, my arms and legs poking out of the door like a deflated jack-in-the-box.

My arms ache. I examine them and notice a dozen or so small, flesh-colored lumps tucked under the skin along my forearms and find patchy discolorations on the underside of my wrists and biceps. The nodes are tender to the touch and the discolorations are the color of plum pulp. I immediately think cancer. Melanoma or blood. Obviously advanced. I rest my forehead against my knees, ass still icy in the freezer, and let the tears come. They never really dry up anymore so I don't even bother to try and stop them. When Shawn, a bakery regular, comes into the shop and finds me swollen-eyed and half-frozen, he slowly backs away and says, "Don't worry. I'll come back."

He returns a few hours later with a smoothie filled with spinach and apples.

"I figured you needed some fruit and vegetables after eating cupcakes all day," he says with a kind smile. Shawn is a leather-wearing punk from Queens with bandolier ammo belts across his chest and rottweiler collars around his neck, like he's straight off the cover of *Anarchy Magazine*. When he's not stomping around the Lower East Side keeping order simply by dressing like he could kick your ass, he runs an urban farm and volunteers at women's shelters, teaching self-defense. He makes himself at home in the bakery and helps himself to a few cupcakes from the display.

"I just noticed this today." I show him my arms.

He pokes at one of the lumps and giggles. "That's awesome! It's like you've got BB pellets underneath your skin. People pay to have that done, you know."

"Is it weird that if it turns out to be something like blood cancer, I don't think I'd bother going through chemo or anything? I feel like it would be a sign. Just be done with this."

"This world is bullshit," Shawn says, lining up Old Fashioned, Dark & Stormy, and White Russian cupcakes in front of him. "But if you did that, who would make me cupcakes?" He shoves all three into his mouth, wrappers and all, and grins at me with overstuffed cheeks. I laugh through watery eyes, my first laugh in weeks.

My business partner arrives at the end of my shift and I tell her I've decided to accept the position on Remote Year. We have a solid team in place, and by the time I leave for Malaysia, there will only be eight months left on a lease neither of us wants to renew. When I first floated Remote Year by her, she seemed pleased at the potential of running the bakery alone. But something shifted and now, we fight.

About what? Five years of perceived inequality, mostly. The details don't matter since inequality is always guaranteed. We are all born with the same natural right to breathe air and take up space on this Earth, but that's where equality ends. We are not born into equality of ambition or intellect or talent or resources, which means there's always something to fight about. We fight long and deep, about who sacrificed what and who brought more to the table when.

"I've been carrying this business for the last two and a half years," she seethes.

"And I carried it for the first two and a half, so now we're even," I snap.

With that, we're done. We both know this is the beginning of a long end. The nodes in my arms throb with the force of my racing heart.

That night, while I walk Buffy, I call my mother and tell her about the lumps.

"My intuition is that this is stress," she says right away. "I mean, go to the dermatologist and get it checked out, but I don't think this is cancer or anything serious. I'm not feeling any sick energy from you. If anything, you sound different. You sound better. Hold on, honey. I'm walking the dog too and Luigi just pooped."

Luigi has the worst timing. I wait, frustrated, for my mother to come back to the phone. As soon as I hear her soft voice come back into my ear, I burst with one hasty breath. "How in the hell do I sound better? I've been crying nonstop for a month. I'm crying right now. If I'm not crying, I'm so angry I lock myself in my apartment because all I want to do is go out and throw things like Dad used to do. I literally ripped one of his shirts off my back the other day because I just couldn't take it anymore. One of those thick Sturgis shirts he wore all the time. Then I tore it into pieces like I was dismembering a body."

"Good," she says. "Get it out. It's just a shirt."

Just thinking about the damn shirt brings back the blind rage, so I jump up and down and stomp both feet into the cement until the force of the earth takes the energy from my bones and sends back a jolt of grounding throbs up through my spine and into my head.

"You taught me to deal with him, you know," my mother says. "Remember in the old house, how the family room was connected to the garage and you could hear him banging around in there at all hours? You were about two and a half, three years old. You learned the alphabet by watching *Wheel of Fortune*. I don't know why I wasn't with you, but when I heard him yelling, I came running down the stairs because I was so shaken up and thought you would be too. You were just sitting there, watching Vanna White turn letters around with all this awful banging around us. You looked at me and said, matter-of-factly, 'Daddy's having a tantrum again.' Then you turned back to *Wheel of Fortune* and asked to buy a vowel. I thought to myself, my three-year-old can handle his outbursts better than I can. After that, I just rolled my eyes. A tantrum."

My mother and I walk in silence for a moment, next to each other despite the thousands of miles between us. I know she is telling me this story to help me feel better. But all it does is confirm what I fear to be true: My father let rage rule his life, and now it rules mine, too.

"What do you mean 'I sound different'?" I ask.

She doesn't answer for a moment, and I can tell she's searching for the right words to convey something that cannot be explained. "It's like the tone of your voice has changed. There's more inflection. You sound like *you*. Like the way you used to sound, before the meds."

"If this is what it feels like to be me, I can't . . . "

"Honey, you call me almost every night when you walk Buffy, so what, six, seven years? You've always sounded so . . . flat. I could always tell if you'd had a few drinks because you sounded up, but this is different. Yesterday when you called because you couldn't sleep, you almost sounded good. Like there was a lightness I hadn't heard in your voice since you were a kid."

"I went and bought some watercolors and brushes yesterday. I don't know what I'm doing, but I also don't know what else to do with myself. Apparently, I don't sleep when I'm not on the Effexor. And the TV is too loud. Too much input."

"Do you know how long it's been since I've heard you talk about doing something creative?" my mother says. "You're an artist at heart, Brooke. You always have been. You're coming back to who you are."

"That was just an hour or two. The rest of the time I'm still depressed and angry. What if that's who I am?"

"Remember a few years ago, when you were at home in Reno and you crawled into bed with me and told me you thought there was something permanently wrong with you? Like you were born broken?"

"Yeah," I sigh.

"I've known you since before you were born. There's always been some anger in you. You came in with it, and it's part of what you need to learn here. But you also came in with light, with the most sensitive and kind heart. Like when I lost my wedding ring when you were four and I was so upset you brought me your little plastic ring with an elephant on it. That little soul is still in there, somewhere."

I sniffle into the phone and want to pull her to me.

"When do you have your follow-up with the psychiatrist?" she asks.

"Tomorrow."

"Call me after your appointment. Keep going. Paint something. I love you."

"I love you too."

I go home and paint late into the night, with deep pools of color that won't dry until morning. Bright magentas, oranges, and yellows leap off the canvas and clash against my blood-red and black furniture. I know when I see Dr. Chin tomorrow, I will need to tell her I want to get off the Wellbutrin. Even though my arms throb and my skin burns and most of the time I feel like I've fallen so deep into myself that I still hold tight to the little voice whispering, *you can make this stop, if you just take one*, I also know I've never noticed color like this before. And I want to hold onto it. I need it. I need color like I need air.

I think of that color when the elevator opens into Dr. Chin's waiting room and I am engulfed in dingy gray walls and dim fluorescent light. I look for the plant, but it's gone, replaced by a coat rack.

"Your appointment was on Tuesday," the receptionist tells me as she checks her handwritten schedule.

It is Thursday.

I pull out my phone and double-check my calendar. According to my schedule, I am here on the right day at the right time. No one called me to confirm, but then again, I didn't confirm either.

"Well shit," I tell her. "This is what I have on my schedule and we didn't confirm ahead of time, so I don't know who screwed up, but here I am."

The receptionist purses her lips and glares at me.

"Okay, have a seat and I'll call Dr. Chin. She's finishing up with someone, so I'll see what she wants to do."

I thank her and plop down in a nearby chair, laughing at the absurdity of this five-star psychiatric experience. I know there must be halfway decent doctors out there, but I seem to have no luck finding them. Or maybe they're just not covered by my insurance.

While I wait for Dr. Chin, the pharmacy leaves an automated message on my phone to tell me my prescriptions are ready for pickup. I cancelled the delivery, but apparently, they filled the script anyway. I wonder how long they would have to sit there before an actual pharmacist picked up the phone. Neither my pharmacist nor Dr. Chin know about the blood in the streets or the shirts ripped off my back or the lumps in my arms. They don't know about the late-night painting or the raindrops on my skin or the subtle changes in my voice. How could they? They wouldn't recognize me if we passed each other on the street.

A few minutes later, Dr. Chin barrels in from around the corner and finds me in the waiting room.

"You missed your appointment on Tuesday," she says, standing over me.

"It was on my calendar for today."

She kneels on the floor next to my chair and starts to say something about scheduling another appointment, but I interrupt her. "It's okay. We don't need to do that. I just wanted to tell you I'm going off the Wellbutrin. I've made it this far without the Effexor, and you said the side effects of getting off it would be way worse than the Wellbutrin."

We lock eyes.

"All right. I guess." Dr. Chin uses the armrest of my chair to push herself up, looks around the waiting room, and casts a "call if there's a problem" in my general direction before walking away.

I spring off the plastic chair and skip into the elevator, ripping the security name tag off my shirt as soon as I reach the lobby. I know I will never see or hear from Dr. Chin again. There is nothing left for her to do if she's not handing me a prescription. As I pass through the security turnstiles and give the guards a little nod, the building's gold revolving doors seem more brilliant than before. I run my fingers across their glimmering frame, waiting for a break in the bodies that go round and round. My time here, in this building, in this city, in this life, is almost up. Like the revolving doors in front of me, I can move in only one direction. There is only one way out of this place: forward. All I can do is push through, pick up speed, and emerge into the blinding Manhattan sun.

7

Two weeks after my appointment with Dr. Chin, I decide I'm ready to stop taking the Wellbutrin. I rearrange my medicine cabinet to mark the occasion. First Aid up top. Prescriptions on the bottom. Sucralfate, isotretinoin, and the two strengths of Levothyroxine on the left. Effexor XR and Wellbutrin XL on the right. A tub of vaseline in the middle, sticky Switzerland in this pharmaceutical war. I can't bring myself to get rid of the antidepressants even though I'm not taking them. I need to know they're there. In case of emergency. In case of desperation. In case the floor falls away.

I fill my mouth with water from the faucet and work my way from the left, swallowing one capsule at a time. When I hit the Vaseline, I smear it over my lips to soothe the peeled and cracked side effects caused by isotretinoin, then close the medicine cabinet and leave.

At the bakery, I brush my arm against the edge of a hot sheet pan, and my skin screams. Normally, I barely notice the sting of a hot pan or the splash of scalding grease. This is different. I wince and cradle my arm against my apron, waiting for the pain to pass, but it pulses like a hornet's sting buried under my skin.

The pain brings a wave of nausea and dizziness, and I sit on a bench near our front entrance with my head between my knees. My burned arm hangs limp by my side, throbbing despite a rational, calm conversation I have with myself.

Shit, this hurts.

But I'm not crying! For once.

A burn has hurt never this much before.

It's just a damn burn. Get back to work. You're being dramatic.

I have never once quit working because of a burn. A cut, maybe. But only to stop the bleeding. One of the worst cuts I ever had was from an oyster knife that slipped and sliced me from thumb to index finger, in the middle of a Saturday dinner rush at the French restaurant I worked in when I was just out of culinary school. I shoved my sliced hand under cold, running water to slow the bleeding and used my good hand to throw the knife into a bucket of bleach water, dump the oyster, and gather a stack of paper towels while the rest of the kitchen clamored on, oblivious. I wrapped a few paper towels around the cut, doubled up on latex gloves, and started shucking again without missing a ticket. Even then, I didn't feel much pain, just the thump of my pulse drumming through my veins.

But burns don't bleed. So why stop?

"Your arms look terrible," my mother always says whenever we manage to find a few days together. "If I didn't know better, I'd think you were hurting yourself." She doesn't understand that the worse my arms look, the more pride I feel. My burns brand me as a person who can withstand anything, announcing to the world without me having to say a word that I am damn tough because I burn myself for a living. Don't fuck with me.

Except it was all a lie. Now I know for sure. Pride may be armor, but apparently the antidepressants were too, because this burn fucking hurts.

The pain radiates out from a thin, inch-long sear, red-hot and bubbling. When I get home that afternoon, I do something I've never done before: take care of the burn. It is still tender to the touch, and I focus on the pain when I reach for the bandages on the top shelf of the medicine cabinet, purposely distracting myself from the untouched antidepressants.

My eyes water as I dab the Neosporin around the wound. I fight back a flood of tears, willing myself to get through this day without collapsing into an inconsolable heap. I need a day, just one, that teeters on the edge of normal long enough to convince me one day can become two. As I wrap my arm in gauze, a warm choke tightens in my throat and my mind tells me to slam my arm into the bathroom wall, over and over, until the acute sting spreads into an all-encompassing ache.

Delete!

I command my mind to stop the image, to erase it from my thoughts. For a moment, it rests, and then sends my arm smacking into the sink again.

Delete!

It shows me wrapping the gauze tighter and tighter.

Delete!

My veins pop and my wrist and hand turn black.

Delete! Delete! Delete!

My good hand pounds my bare thigh like a gavel in a cacophonous courtroom. When I come back from wherever I just went, I realize I've hit myself hard enough to bruise.

I turn back to the burn and finish dressing it with a delicate touch despite my shaking hands. *Let me be through the worst of it,* I beg, exhausted from the horror reels spinning through my head. I realize I've forgotten to shower. I'm covered in bakery and nausea sweat, and for all I know, I just sealed a damp cluster of bacteria into an open wound. In a blink I see my arm, oozing and infected. I see the burn necrotized around the edges and streaks of black creeping in all directions. I see a hospital bed I can't afford and a flurry of doctors whizzing around me and an arm that can't be saved because of one dumb mistake.

In a breath, the shower. Gauze balled up on the floor by the toilet. Fire water running over the burn. Head between my legs. Holding back a howl.

I hold the howl in through another dressing, through the afternoon and into the night, while I make a long list of everything I need to do before leaving New York in 124 days. I need to buy a suitcase, close my PO box, cancel *Food & Wine Magazine*, get extra passport photos, eat a bagel and lox, book flights, figure out where exactly Malaysia is on a map.

I hold the howl in as the days pass, while I begin to arrange the logistical things like vaccinations, visas, and documents. I hold it in while I think through the complicated things like working my way around the condo board's prohibition on subletters, finding a remote job, and figuring out how taxes work when you're traveling around the world.

I hold in the howl while I push away the terrifying things: the terrorism clause on my international insurance, the biopsy results from the lumps in my arm, the Zika outbreak ravaging Central and South America. I even hold it in while I avoid the heartbreaking things: saying goodbye to Buffy, giving up the bakery, leaving my home.

And then I get an email:

> Congratulations! I am delighted to tell you that you have made it to the final level of casting for *CHOPPED*. Your *CHOPPED* competition date in New York City is set for June 22.

That's when I lose it. I howl with such force that capillaries burst in the puffs of skin under my eyes. Bubbles of snot coat my keyboard as I sob into my laptop while wondering why in the hell the producers chose me for a cooking competition when all I know about anymore is cupcakes and frosting, neither of which takes any real culinary mastery. Mix wet into dry. Beat butter and sugar. Don't burn shit.

I howl at the thought of responding to the producers with my tail between my legs, embarrassed to have interviewed before I got off the antidepressants, only to back out. I howl at the thought of going through with filming. I will be forced into a lie, forced into representing myself as if I am successful, when in reality I am crumbling. I think of cutting myself in the middle of the competition and bleeding all over the set.

This is too much. All of it.

I call my mother, my eyes so swollen from crying that the numbers on phone screen blur into a white blob.

"This is about freezing up on the diving board," she says.

"The diving board?"

"Remember, it was your senior year in college and you'd already hit the qualifying score for Nationals five or six times, but you had to do it at Regionals to officially qualify. And my mother had just died so I was a mess in the stands. We were both so sad your dad wasn't there because he would have been so proud. There was a lot of pressure. You kept changing your dive lineup and you wouldn't listen to your coach. She finally gave up. Then you balked on a dive and your ponytail braid hit the board so hard that everyone thought you hit your head. I remember you were so embarrassed you came and stayed in the hotel room with me instead of staying with your team."

"Obviously I remember because it was terrible. What does that have to do with this?" Goddamnit my mother can be annoying when she's trying to get to the point.

"You know how to cook just like you knew how to dive." My mother says, punctuating her point by pouring herself a bowl of smoked almonds. The crackling sound of the bag of nuts grates through the phone speaker and into my eardrums.

"But that was a dinky college diving meet no one cared about. This is national television."

"It's the same situation, just a different manifestation." I hear her clunk the cabinets, open and close the fridge, run the faucet.

"So why would I put myself in the same situation?"

"Because it's giving you an opportunity to heal the wound so this pattern doesn't show up in your life again. It's going to keep showing up until you deal with it."

I want to throw my phone at the wall. So many of our conversations end up here, with my mother giving me her best, well-intentioned directions to her Woo Woo World while I bang my head against the "No Trespassing" sign at each road's entrance.

"This is going to sound really weird," she continues. "Like it's way out there. But I heard this guy on the radio the other day. Alan Somethingorother. He's kind of a spiritual counselor, and he works with people one-on-one. I heard him do a short facilitation with someone who called into the show and it was so powerful. I could feel the shift in energy for this person. It's all based on self-compassion."

"I'm sorry, what? Also, can you stop eating? All I can hear is you crunching into the phone."

"Sorry, honey," she says. "You know me. I'm having almonds for dinner. Anyway, at the end of the show, Alan offered listeners a one-off session, so I booked an appointment and talked with him yesterday. The session was recorded so I can send it to you if you want to see what it's like. You'll have to put up with listening to your mother cry, but only because it was so effective. I'm telling you, this is powerful stuff."

I imagine my mother standing in the kitchen in her pink, fuzzy robe and slippers, neck and shoulder scrunching the phone in place. Fingers covered in almond salt, she's waiting for me to dismiss her platitudes, waiting for me to tell her this depression, this anger, beats as steady as my heart and no amount of self-compassion can stop the pulse. But after two months of antidepressant withdrawal and fifteen years of this, I am sick of that beat. Sick of myself. Sick of the self-pity. Sick of the tears, the wading around in my own shit, the open window.

"You can send it to me, but I'm not making any promises," I tell her.

My mother emails me a link to Alan's website and her session. I don't listen to the recording. Not yet, anyway. It's all too much for today. Instead I surf Alan's site. It is splashed in blues and littered with buzzwords—awakening, detox, karma—with promises of breakthroughs in money, love, and career. *Bullshit*, I think. The therapeutic equivalent of late-night detergent infomercials claiming to remove stubborn stains from any fabric, even caked on grease and blood. Thirty days of using our secret formula to make your clothes look like new! Thirty days of karma detox to scrub your soul clean!

What if the soul is too shattered to scrub? If, over the years, it disintegrates layer by layer until there is nothing left? What then? How do karma or crystals or compassion cleanse something that no longer exists? People always talk about how antidepressants flatten a person, how they push the issues down and dull it away. But people are wrong. I was never numb. I was simply not here. And now that it's time to let my soul back in, I find all the places that are broken. What is even left of me to recover?

~~~~~~~~~~~~~

When the morning light peeks over the buildings outside my window and warms my skin, I notice I am weightless, somehow, as if the darkness of yesterday has faded away with the bitter cold winds of spring. I don't wake with dread or the familiar body aches and lingering nausea of the past few weeks and months. I feel like I can go spend the day with my friends, on Governor's Island like we planned, and drink cold beer in newly hung hammocks without wondering if I might break into sobs if I knock a beer into the grass. I actually look forward to spending the day in the world, and to hear the call of birds instead of traffic.

This is new.

Maybe I don't need Alan and his self-compassion at all, I think. *All the withdrawal symptoms came on so fast, maybe they stop suddenly too.*

I curl up on the couch, feeling this strange, calm energy I've awoken with. It seems like a switch was activated in the night and has sent me into this day with a new mind. Whoever this woman is, I like her. I am curious about her. She sips her coffee without needing to turn on the TV or check her phone. She swirls the creamy, hot liquid in her mouth and notices as her taste buds light up with notes of toffee and tangerine and smoke. She thinks about what she might do if coffee appears in a *Chopped* basket. Desserts are obvious—coffee and chocolate, coffee and cherry, coffee and caramel. Any one of those combinations could be folded into ice cream, whisked into custard, or whipped into frosting. But before the dessert round, she must make it through the appetizers and entrées. Coffee is trickier then. Not impossible, but it takes some finesse to keep the perfect coffee-rubbed rib eye from tasting like a steak that fell into a bucket of Folgers.

I throw on an old sweater, but the rough, synthetic fibers irritate my skin. I've worn this sweater for years, but suddenly I can't stand it so I toss it over the back of a chair and decide it will be the first thing in the giveaway pile once I start cleaning out my apartment. The sweater is cheap and ugly anyway. It's also boxy and heavy and its knit pattern reminds me of the gnarled, orange and vomit-green carpet that once lined a house my father built in the '80s. Everything in that house was a patchwork mess. My father was colorblind and couldn't pick red out of a green lineup. So he mixed leftover paint together, from all corners of the rainbow, and slathered it across the walls. Never mind that the rest of us got dizzy when we walked in the front door or that the carpet was so coarse it burned my knees red and raw when I played on the floor.

Fuck that carpet. And the sweater.

The tranquility of the past few minutes drops out of me in an instant and I stomp over to my kitchen, pull a garbage bag out of the cabinet, and stuff the sweater into the bag as the prickles of rage greet me.

No, no, no, I think. *Go back. Go back. Go back to her.*

I am so tired of this shit.

It occurs to me to move this energy, to channel this budding anger into something else, so I grab another garbage bag and bring both of them into my bedroom. I grab clothes I never wear and stuff them one after the other into the bag with the sweater until the bag is stretched and barely knots at the top. Then I walk to the bathroom and go through the cabinets, throwing out half-empty bottles of toiletries, samples of perfume, and old hair clips left over from high school. I make my way from one cabinet to the other until I get to the last one, the one over the sink.

The familiar row of orange bottles greets me, still meticulously arranged from left to right. They are mocking me, each bottle filled with thirty individual monuments to the ghost of my father, my business, the life I am trying to leave.

No more.

The contents of the bottles rattle as I grab the containers in one handful and heave them into the garbage bag. Then I grab the prescription slip for Prozac, crumple it into a ball, and throw it away with the rest. Even amid rage and exhaustion, I know I will never take that drug. It doesn't matter if it might ease the symptoms. It doesn't matter if prescribing Prozac to "bridge" between drugs is common practice. It doesn't matter if it is against a doctor's recommendations. It doesn't matter if it is an industrial-strength, stupid decision. I simply cannot bring myself to throw another drug into my system, to return to the scene of the crime and risk smearing blood around after weeks of trying to clear the evidence.

I gather the bag by the top corners and twirl it into a knot as I march toward the front door of my apartment. For a brief moment, I panic.

What if my hair starts falling out in clumps again? Or my stomach turns to fire? Or my face breaks out with bloody pustules?

I drop the bag in the middle of the kitchen and dig until I find the package of Isotretinoin that keeps my face clear. I pull it out and fling it over my shoulder and it lands on the floor with a smack. Isotretinoin is expensive, a few hundred dollars for thirty capsules. Everything else is cheap, generic. Easy to refill in the event of internal revolt.

I knot the bag again and stomp to the garbage room across the hall, barefoot. The room smells like sour milk and stale air freshener, and the floor sticks to my feet. The heavy, steel door shuts behind me and when it clicks closed I know I am alone and I stuff the bag into the chute and scream one long "fuck" into the room. My voice echoes off the tiled walls as the bag clunks down the metal gutter. I listen to it fall, until somewhere between here and thirty floors below, there is nothing but silence.

I go back to my apartment and put the kettle on for another pot of coffee. While it's heating, I strip down and step into the shower to wash the garbage room off my feet. The bathroom, somehow, feels freer with its empty cabinets and I breathe into its lightness, noting my aching forearms as I scrub between my toes. The kettle squeaks as I turn off the water. I wrap myself in a towel to head to the kitchen, but catch myself in the mirror on the way.

I drop the towel to the ground. Naked, I look at myself in the mirror, analyzing the lines and curves and angles of my body I have inspected for so many years. I am shaped like my mother—petite, with sloping shoulders, a narrow ribcage, and wide hips—but with the muscles and sturdiness of my father, a physical combination I have always found to be aesthetically perplexing, as if Ken's muscles were photoshopped onto Barbie's frame. I use my hands to push back the flesh on my hips, revealing my hipbones and erasing the feminine curves of my pelvis into a beautiful, straight line.

Be less space.

As I release the pinch on my hips and they flop back into the arcs I loathe, I notice the same patchy discolorations on my arms have appeared on my butt, the back of my thighs, and the inside of my right knee. By the time I finish going over each inch of flesh, I've counted more than forty nodules on my body. I am jolted out of my inspection only by the chime of a text message telling me to be ready to leave for Governor's Island in twenty minutes.

I check the once-boiling water in the kettle to find it cool. I lost an hour scanning every inch of my body. The calm woman from this morning is gone, and I panic. It's hot out. I need to find my summer clothes, but I just threw half of them down the garbage chute. When I do find something light, I put it on, but it doesn't fit or it itches and it's just wrong and everything I have is wrong and the more clothes I try on the angrier I get and the angrier I get the more my arms ache. I put on a pair of shorts and then one shirt after another and with each one that doesn't work I throw it into a pile next to another garbage bag filled with everything that used to be right but is now so wrong. I find a flowy shirt that might fit, but it's wrinkled. It's the only summer shirt I have left and I can't wear it if it's wrinkled so I pull my rickety ironing board out from behind a row of coats and set it up and plug in my iron and stand topless in my bedroom, waiting.

The iron steams and I run it across the shirt, but it's too hot and pulls on the delicate fabric and the shirt puckers and I scream at the iron.

I want to put the iron to my skin.

I rip the cord out of the plug and push the iron across the ground to cool down. I pull the shirt off the board and I put it on. The collar chokes me and the fabric is a million little needles and I am too much space. I need to scream. To hit something. To destroy. The bed and pillows are the only safe spot. I can't get to them because the ironing board is in the way. I reach under it to try and free the latch, but it's rusty and stuck.

My vision narrows and I feel the blood pulsing through the lumps in my arms.

Destroy.

I flip the ironing board over and slam it on the ground, legs straight up. I fight with the rods and try to release them from their hold, but they don't move. I jam my foot onto the edge of the board to steady it and grab each leg with one hand and push the legs apart to try to slide them out of place, but they don't move and instead the metal legs bend in half, dislodging parts of the ironing board and sending screws and coils flying across the room. I push and pull at the board until its mechanisms are fully loose and I bend the whole thing into a pile of mangled metal.

It is only in sheer exhaustion that the anger stops.

I fall to the floor, panting. Is this how it felt for my father? Did he throw trash cans and keyboards and hammers at the wall because he needed to physically see the destruction, proof that whatever was inside him was gone and instead scattered across the floor? Did he wonder, like I do, if the anger would ever stop or if it would keep regenerating and grow stronger with each release? Could he feel the anger coming or did he just suddenly, unpredictably, snap? Is this all he gave me? A pair of sturdy legs and a temper strong enough to tear down everything I built? I don't want to live in my father's world. The autopsy listed pancreatic cancer as his cause of death, but maybe it was a lifetime of rage that rotted him from the inside out. But the anger is so immediate, so all encompassing. What other choice did he have? What other choice do I have?

I cave on the floor, next to the mangled ironing board, and remember that I am my mother's daughter, too. Here was a woman who, after being widowed at forty-seven, survived breast cancer, underwent open-heart surgery, kept a business afloat with forty employees during the recession, and did it all while raising an only child with suicidal tendencies. And yet she never succumbed to rage, never lost that sparkle for living. Maybe it is time to do as my mother would do, not as my father did.

I crawl to my laptop, pull it down to the floor, and listen to the recording of my mother and Alan. He guides her to speak to herself with compassion, like she is comforting a little girl who scraped her knee. I've heard this tone from her so many times before, after each of my own bumps and cuts and bruises when she scooped me up, wiped my tears, and dressed the wound with a touch so gentle I barely felt the sting. It never occurred to me that a person could treat themselves with that level of tender care, especially in the company of another adult. But Alan's voice is like a flash of light in a stormy sea, guiding my mother to release a memory I knew had gripped her tight for years. She trusts him with a part of her that had been wounded for so long, and in listening to her strength I decide I could forgive Alan's pithy promises of transformation so long as I am allowed to transform in the safety of my own home. I no longer trust myself not to snap out in the world.

I reach my right hand to the keyboard and with one finger, type an email to Alan, asking for help. Then I text my friend to tell her to head to Governor's Island on her own.

I drop my head back onto the floor, close my eyes, and think of my mother. She always said it's like she was born with the curtain half open, like the barrier between the perceived human experience and the soul's purpose never quite closed. From the time she was little, she says, she could "see" beyond the three-dimensional world in front of her and tap into a level of existence that seems to elude most everyone else. Over the years, this gift has led her to understand the world through a distinct ethereal lens, one that goes beyond the constraints of religious doctrine and constitutional law.

It goes something like this: It is all a game. An eternal game played by eternal beings; a universal Easter egg hunt of sorts, with players who incarnate as humans into this world, again and again, embodying a particular play piece each time. Round and round we go, born into families and cultures telling us the game we're playing is about money and power and fame, separation and segregation and dark versus light. But really, the whole point of the game is to figure out it's a game—a game about discovering we are all one, each of us a spark of the same source.

Clues appear like hidden eggs, my mother says. Little eggs of light that show up through everything from compassion to art to nature to heroic acts.

Reminders of our true identity. Think Buddhism without the whole "life is suffering" bit + Christianity without heaven and hell + a good dose of The Matrix thrown in. But since this is the most difficult game ever created, we begin each hunt blind, deaf, and dumb. Extraordinarily dumb. So dumb we don't even remember we're playing a game, or that there are even any eggs to be found. We rig the game from the start with whatever economic, racial, physical, political, and familial bullshit exists in the sliver of the world we choose for ourselves. We think suffering in a Mombasa slum is different from suffering in a Manhattan high-rise, but pain is pain is pain. We all spend most of our lives just trying to avoid the suffering, occasionally tripping over an egg in our most untethered moments. Still, we often don't realize what we've found until we trip over it a few times. And even then we're not sure because we start to wonder if there are better eggs around.

When we inevitably don't figure out the game at the end of our life—no matter, there's another round right behind it. And another and another and another. As many as it takes. Maybe it's a new scenario, or maybe it's one we've done 1,000 times before. We get to choose, since we have to experience them all in order to understand we are of the same source, just wrapped in different skin.

Besides, we can only win the game together. Only when every last one of us learns to see through the illusion of difference and embodies unconditional love will we all move forward in peace. But this unconditional love cannot exist without all that is ugly and threatening in the world. Because how can we learn unconditional love if we have never felt hatred, disgust, and resentment? Therefore, we've all been the beggar and we've all been filthy rich. We've all been enslaved and we've all cracked the whip. We've all been raped and we've all been the rapist.

Now here we are, after 200,000 years on the merry-go-round of humanity. We have been wounded, all of us. The longer we play the game, the more scar tissue that forms, and this tissue, if not worked through, shows up as pain. Any sort of pain. Rage. Shame. Guilt. Fibromyalgia. Addiction. Poverty. Abuse. Obesity. Cancer. Depression. But since this is all a game, the scars are illusions, carnival-mirror reflections distorting who we really are. We must rid ourselves of the scar tissue, the distraction clouding the vision of our playing fields. As anyone who's ever been injured knows, to work through physical scar tissue on a bum knee is painful. But to work through existential scar tissue of the soul?

Excruciating.

8

"Your intake questionnaire," Alan says on the other end of the phone, where he's calling me from somewhere in Florida, "it's amazing. Fifteen years. That's a big chunk of your life. I'd say it's a breakthrough just getting off the medications. And a trip around the world? And you're going to be on *Chopped*? I love that show!"

"Uh-huh. Yeah." My voice is thin and meek. I am exhausted, slumped over my desk and staring out my window, *the* window, my mind and body raw and torn open.

Alan continues. "The picture I'm getting is you've had this stuff holding your parts together and now you're starting to get off the medications, you don't feel stable because the structure and glue is gone. But now you can rebuild a structure that's you, instead of this giant bandage that's been holding you together for a long time."

There is sureness in Alan's voice, and a distinct lack of pity. I am so used to the mindless routine of doctor's offices, where the only thing distinguishing my chart from the next person's is a grainy photocopy of my ID. Alan has never seen my face. His intake form didn't ask me about my family's history of diabetes or liver disease, but to rate how true the following statement felt to me: "Miracles happen in my life on a regular basis." I rolled my eyes at the question and clicked on the bubble for "not true at all." Then I slammed my laptop shut and tensed every muscle in my body, digging my fingernails into the palms of my hands and clenching my biceps and butt and hamstrings to contain the rage until my body was on fire and my mind was finally clear and all I could feel was pressure.

Miracles are for lottery winners and Jesus freaks and people who wake up from comas. Miracles are not for thirty-year-old white women and their first-world problems.

"What do you think?" Alan asks after a stretch of silence. "Is that true or not true? What does that make you feel?"

I glance at the sketchbook pushed off to my right, open from last night's attempt at painting a pear. Over and over I tried to draw the bulbous fruit, but the charcoal lines never went where they should. And when I went to fill them in with color, the outlines couldn't contain the seeping puddles of green and brown, leaving me with vaguely fruit-shaped blobs the color of rot. Before I answer Alan, I start crying over the pears.

"It's only been two months since getting off the first drug," I tell him, embarrassed by my obvious need for help, by my own weakness, by pears this strange man can't even see. "I didn't see any point of going off them before. I was just waiting to die. But I don't feel like there's an upside of being off the drugs either. I'm tired of crying. Nothing is moving fast enough. Nothing makes any sense. I don't want any of this anymore. Forget Remote Year. Forget *Chopped*. I want out of all of this. Now."

I wait for Alan to tell me some people are just wired differently, that maybe now isn't a good time to get off the drugs, and that he doesn't take health insurance. But instead he lets out a long, soft "mmmhmmm" that sends me melting into my chair. That one sigh of understanding tells me this isn't about tallying up my suffering to rationalize insurance reimbursement. Instead, it's an invisible hand reaching through the phone lines, beckoning me to grab it tight and let myself be pulled to safety.

"My basic worldview is pretty simple," Alan says. "I believe our souls live outside of physical reality, and that the soul knows what is best and perfect for us. Imagine that our fully enlightened soul projects its light through us, like our mind and body is a camera lens. The light goes through the lens and projects a picture of everything that is good or bad in our lives—our job, our health, our relationships. If we don't like the picture, it's because our soul is trying to shine its light through a cracked lens. Instead of getting the things that bring us joy, we get sadness or despair or frustration or anger."

"So what the hell do you actually do about it?" I blurt out, feeling like this banter is all well and good in concept, but wondering how it translates into reality.

"We look at what's going on with your life and we see things that don't feel good to you. That gives us information. Our soul, our consciousness, projects our world and reveals our experience. Whether our soul's light is clear or distorted is the primary cause of things that either make us happy or don't make us happy."

Bullshit.

I don't understand how my soul is causing these problems when it seems pretty fucking clear my problems are rooted in everything from my toxic business partnership to antidepressant withdrawal to a dead father who managed to both love me and smash my jack-o-lantern while I was out trick-or-treating. And what about real problems like single-use plastic and poverty and corruption and racism and terrorism?

"I'm sorry, Alan," I say, frustrated. "I just don't get how you fix all this."

"We fix it by focusing inward and giving ourselves compassion. That clears the distorted lens and lets our soul's light shine through in its full strength. When that happens, we get some magical outcomes in our life. I don't know how much you're into this spiritual stuff. Does any of this sound consistent with what you see and believe?"

Logically this makes about as much sense to me as confessing your sins to a stranger in a box who tells you to solve your problems by chanting a few poems over a beaded necklace.

I push back. "I've never believed in the whole bearded-man-in-a-white-robe-in-the-sky thing. But what about the whole adage about putting up with suffering because it's your cross to bear or what you need in order to grow as a human? Or about learning from the hard times and finding the silver lining? You know, all that greeting-card bullshit."

The tone in Alan's voice changes from lullaby-soft to confident and bold.

"I don't buy into those spiritual teachings," he says. "When people can't figure out how to fix their life, they have to make sense of it so their brain doesn't break and they don't jump out of the window."

This statement stops me cold. Alan doesn't know about the window, about the 5.58 seconds. Yet in five minutes he has somehow drilled into the single greatest choice of my life: to live or to leave. I adjust my eyes and gaze at the windowpane, and the skyline blurs as my reflection comes into focus. I see the edges of myself etched into the window, the edges of someone who chose, on that cold December night, to live. And that choice led me here, on the phone with a stranger in Florida.

Alan continues. "My belief is that we go piece-by-piece. We examine the broken piece, heal it with our own compassion, and put the fixed piece back in. Then we take another piece, we pull it out, and we work with it. Eventually there becomes a cumulative benefit, an acceleration process, like putting a puzzle together."

Something about what Alan says feels true, even though I don't entirely understand it. Maybe he has something to offer me. Maybe it's time to stop fighting. To listen. To try.

Or maybe I just want it to be true because he makes it all sound so simple. Or maybe I'm just desperate. Probably both.

"I'd love to believe it's possible, but I haven't seen any evidence of it in my own life at this point. And I have no idea what you mean by 'compassion.'"

"Do you want to give the process a try and see if we can cut the intensity of whatever you're feeling right now? All you have to do is say a few phrases out loud right after me," Alan says.

"Okay," I say, too drained to work through the mental gymnastics of understanding this process. It's easier just to surrender, to go with whatever he says.

"Don't overthink it. Just pour the *feeling* of compassion into all the wounded parts of you that need healing while you do it, okay?"

"Okay." I think back to my mother's own call with Alan, and how she spoke to herself with the same tender tone of love and care she always used for me. I try to feel her, channel her, imitate her.

"Just repeat the following statement after me," Alan says. "'I'm so sorry you can't stop crying.'"

"I'm so sorry you can't stop crying," I say. It is strange to hear my voice saying these words. I am self-conscious, somehow, of speaking out loud to myself.

"I'm so sorry everything is so messed up," Alan says.

"I'm so sorry everything is so messed up," I repeat. I feel like time has slowed for a moment, like, in just repeating the phrase, I give myself permission to acknowledge that yes, there are bigger problems in the world, but my little world has issues too.

"I'm so sorry you feel trapped." My chest tightens, and I notice how with each repeated phrase I seem to have a physical response. "I'm so sorry you don't feel safe in your body." My eyes tear. "I'm so sorry your emotions are overwhelming." My throat burns.

"How do you feel now?" Alan asks after a pause.

"Shitty. Like everything you said is true. I don't understand where you're getting these statements."

"We're not necessarily focusing on reality. We're focusing on how you *perceive* reality."

"So how do you know what to say?" I ask.

"We look at how you're feeling or what you notice when certain statements come up," Alan says. "If there's a big emotional reaction, or maybe a big physical reaction, it usually means we're onto a big issue. So we focus on what we can feel. Did you see anything in your mind's eye or feel anything in your body while you were saying those last statements?"

"My throat, I guess. It's like everything just sticks in the bottom of my throat, you know? Like it all wells up right there. I feel like I'm a kid trying not to cry over spilled milk. I know I shouldn't be upset about it, but I am. It's ridiculous."

"It's not ridiculous," Alan says. "Let's do a little more. Repeat after me, this time pouring compassion into your throat, to the part of you that feels like a little kid: I'm so sorry you're scared."

For a moment, I pause. I don't know where this statement comes from, or the fear he's referring to. But I decide not to interrupt, not to question. I follow directions and say, "I'm so sorry you're scared," and focus on my throat. An image begins to form in my mind's eye, a long-forgotten memory. I am very small. My eyes just meet the edge of my mother's bathroom counter.

"I'm so sorry they wouldn't just listen to you," Alan continues, and I follow.

My mother is in the room with me.

"I'm so sorry it hurts so much inside."

Something has happened here.

"I'm so sorry they made you feel wrong for having deep and difficult feelings."

My little knuckles grip around the barrel of a wooden hairbrush.

"I'm so sorry they wouldn't let you scream as much as you wanted to."

I smash the head of the hairbrush against the porcelain counter

"I'm so sorry you didn't know what to do with those feelings."

I bang it over and over and over again.

75

"I'm so sorry your feelings made others uncomfortable too."

"This is not how we act," my mother says and stomps out of the room.

"I'm so sorry they forced you to swallow your feelings."

My mother returns and upturns my piggy bank on the floor.

"I'm so sorry those feelings got trapped in your body and never left."

You are going to pay for the hairbrush.

"I'm so sorry something terrible became even worse because of how they dealt with it."

Nickels and dimes all scattered about.

My mother's bathroom fades from my mind's eye and I am back in my apartment, stunned by this long-forgotten memory and Alan's ability to pull it out of me a half hour into our first phone call.

"How do your chest and throat feel now?" Alan asks.

"Like it could burst any second with anger and rage. I just want to be like my father and throw things and scream and tell people they're fucking idiots and not care about the consequences."

"Yep." Alan's voice is soothing, without a trace of judgment. "Was either one of his parents like that, too?"

"My grandfather was, I'm told, but he died when I was three so I don't remember. I just know he had a terrible temper and once threw my dad into a burning fireplace, but I don't know much beyond that."

"What if this rage is passed down, and you're paying the price for things up your family tree you didn't even know about? It's like this inherited scream has been getting passed down through generations, and now it's stuck inside of you."

This statement cuts through my chest and I don't respond, not because it feels untrue, but because it feels so true and obvious I can't believe it's never occurred to me.

"I think if we could clear out some anger, it would be a huge sigh of relief for you."

"Okay," I say, knowing this won't fix everything. But somehow this whole process feels significant, like whatever we're doing matters.

"Take a breath and repeat after me: I'm so sorry it's not safe to scream."

I fall asleep for hours after I get off the phone with Alan. It's dark when I wake, and my limbs are heavy with emotional sludge. Buffy peed on the carpet and, when I discover the spot, she puts her ears back and hides under the bed. She knows she did something wrong and my heart breaks for her because it's not her fault. When I try to lure her out from under the bed, she growls. I let her be, and it's not until after midnight that she emerges and paws at my feet for a walk.

Manhattan is as dark as it gets. Shadows of people crossing the street stretch long into the night. Lights from all the windows stack one on top of the other, twinkling toward the sky in manufactured constellation. Buffy sniffs a Callery tree, lifts a leg, looks at me. I wonder what she was thinking when I was on the phone with Alan, if I scared her, if I somehow hurt her, if she even noticed.

I think of the three worlds in New York City—on the street, underground, and in the skyscrapers—millions of realities tucked into boxes thirty stories high and packed into subway cars thirty feet below. In the rising towers, a baby is born just as someone else takes a final breath. One couple fights and another makes love for the first time. Underground, tens of thousands of others pour in and out of the subway, digesting their troubles as they move through the belly of New York. And yet, standing on this Manhattan street, I am alone. Just like everyone else.

Buffy and I turn on to Lexington Avenue. It's quiet tonight. Eerie. No sirens in the distance. No horns from impatient drivers with nowhere to go. This sort of quiet usually comes only twice a year: after the sun sets on Christmas Day, and on the first evening snowfall of the year. It shouldn't be like this right now, and the stillness makes me uneasy. I take a deep breath and exhale with a shallow huff. My heart rate ticks up, and I close my eyes to shake the silence.

Only anger comes.

Suddenly, I am aware of how little peace and stillness I have had in my eight years in Manhattan, how the antidepressants masked the now-obvious fact that this city, this business, this life, was wrong for me. And I am fucking pissed off. The questions come at me again, one after the other.

If my whole New York City life isn't right for me, what else in my life went wrong? Would I have become a chef if the first time I burned myself I actually felt the pain? Would I have actually planned for a future? Would I have even wanted one?

The rage builds in my limbs and my arms are on fire and I breathe faster, faster. I know I need to get back to my apartment because I am going to blow and I'm in public and that's not okay and it's not safe here so I pick up the pace and turn the corner down 38th Street. The bumps in my arms are pulsing and I want to shave off my skin and my brain is rattled but there's nothing I can do to stop it and I am tired, so tired. *What if this never gets better and for the rest of my life I'm okay one moment and not okay the next and there's no way to predict it and it's not okay to live like this and this is what the drugs are for and if this is how I will be without them then I need to get back on them because I can't live in this world.*

I walk into the middle of 38th Street and stop in the darkness on a small patch of asphalt where the streetlamps don't shine. In this spot, I am part of the night. I look around and gasp for air. All around me, above and below, people live their lives, but I can't see them and I can't hear them. I am the night.

A pair of headlights glow in the distance, waiting for the stoplight to turn. Long shadows flicker just outside my gaze.

Before I realize what I'm doing, my lungs pack with air and I'm screaming so loud and long and pure that the city stops around me as the scream echoes through the street. It starts low in my lungs and raises in pitch until it trickles out thin and piercing. I feel all life on the block suspend for a moment, looking for the source of the sound. But they cannot see me. I am hidden in plain sight in the shadows of the night.

Buffy pulls at her leash and we walk, as the world looks on and wonders.

9

Ninety-three days until I arrive in Malaysia. Eighty-eight days without Effexor XR. Fifty-one days without Wellbutrin. Twenty-seven days until *Chopped* films.

I am a pebble of fury tucked into the pocket of a slingshot. Every stubbed toe, smashed cupcake, and travel document pulls the elastic back just a little more until the tension is all too much and the pebble hurls itself through space and blows a boulder-sized hole through the wall.

I burn a pot of onions and scream. I fumble with the plastic on a package of batteries and scream. Buffy pees on the floor and I scream. Her little body shakes when I come into the room. I did this to her. I break both our hearts every time I wail and she cowers. So I take her to Dolores and let her stay there, in peace. I come back to my apartment and, as I clean up her urine, I scream.

When I get on the phone with Alan a week later, he wastes no time. "Go ahead and take a nice, full breath," he says. "Focus on your heart center: I'm so sorry you're angry."

"I'm so sorry you're angry," I say out loud, my voice quivering through tears.

"I'm so sorry your father's anger found a home in you."

I clench my fists.

"I'm so sorry your grandfather's anger found a home in you."

My forearms cramp.

"I'm so sorry the main thing you got from them was anger."

I want to hit something.

"I'm so sorry you inherited a family curse."

Punish myself.

"I'm so sorry you don't know how to get the anger out."

I close my eyes and see a forest.

"I'm so sorry it's been like this since before you remembered."

The fog hangs low and gray.

"I'm so sorry no one can help you."

Fires burn all around.

"I'm so sorry you're not in control of your emotions or your life."

Each one sending streams of suffocating smoke to the sky.

"I'm so sorry you can't stop the pain."

The fires roar.

Alan pauses and takes a breath.

"How do you feel or what are you thinking about?" he asks.

I know my body is in New York, at my desk. The small of my back sticks to my leather chair. Someone shuffles to the elevator just outside my apartment door. Water runs through the pipes in the wall. I am here. Grounded in a high-rise. Yet a part of me is out there, in a flaming forest I know I've never been to. For a moment I am scared to tell Alan what I see, what I feel. What if it's nonsense? What if he doesn't understand it? I don't even understand it. But there is something about doing this over the phone that allows me to let my guard down in a way I've never been able to do in front of a traditional therapist.

"I see fires everywhere," I tell him, the images of forest fires whirling in my head. "My throat is raw and my jaw is throbbing. This fire, this scene, feels so real. It's me, but it's not me. It's like being in a waking dream."

"Can you tell me a little more about what this sort of waking dream feels like?" Alan asks, no trace of judgment in his voice.

I open my eyes, see my reflection again against the windowpane.

"You know how when you take a long drive, one that takes you beyond the city limits, and the radio station begins to crackle?"

"When you enter into a new radio frequency? Yeah, I understand," Alan says.

"When you drive miles away from one radio tower and toward the signal of another, the music begins to change. Bits of country twang break the beat of classic rock. You are still driving the car, in full control of your surroundings and destination. Only the music around you changes, the country crooning overtaking a power ballad, a few notes at a time. Once you get closer to the country signal the whole station flips, but you are still driving, still in control, just as you were before. It's like that."

"So when we do the statements, it's like we're driving on a loop together and just waiting to see what new radio stations come through?" Alan asks.

"Right, but it's like I can also turn off the radio and my mind would be back in my apartment, with jackhammers blaring outside and Buffy curled up at my feet. Does that make sense?"

"It does," Alan says. "Who knows what you're tapping into. This forest, it could be connected to a past life. Like you're remembering something that on some level you've experienced."

I pause at the suggestion, the truth of that reality feeling too big and overwhelming to consider. Maybe my over-active imagination is just flowing in and out of a dream-like state. Maybe my brain is creating a series of metaphors to help rationalize its adjustment into unmedicated equilibrium. Maybe I am tapping into something bigger than this world. I don't know. I can't ever truly know. I decide it doesn't matter, and to simply leave the radio dial in my mind untouched whenever I began to utter the phrase "I'm so sorry." Whatever images emerge in my mind's eye seem to be some sort of message from my subconscious. I commit to feeling every aspect of the mental images, letting them appear so clear in my mind that if I had the artistic ability to render the scene in photorealistic detail, I could sketch it out down to the pixel.

"I suppose anything is possible," I say.

"Let's keep going with this," Alan says.

I close my eyes and let the radio dial crackle, the forest returning to my mind's eye. As the image fills my head, my throat begins to tighten, as if I were in the middle of this forest, inhaling the smoke.

"I'm so sorry you can't put out the fire."

I put one fire out. Two new ones start.

"I'm so sorry they come back in the same or different form."

The process never ends.

"I'm so sorry when you thought the battle was won, it wasn't."

It is not possible to win.

"I'm so sorry there's fire under the ground everywhere, waiting to sprout up."

It doesn't matter which way I go.

"I'm so sorry there is no good and right direction."

There's no way out of this place.

"I'm so sorry whichever way you go, you'll suffer."

No one comes to the rescue.

"I'm so sorry no one came back for you."

Embers burn all around me.

"I'm so sorry you didn't know what you did to deserve this."

Fires suffocated, but never extinguished.

"I'm so sorry you can't trust the ground you walk on."

I want to fan the smoke away, but I know the fire still burns underneath. I let the smoke consume me. I let it fill my lungs and burn my throat and with each cry my breath gets longer and longer until I surrender to the smoke and drift into the darkness. Suddenly the fires extinguish and I feel a rush of warm energy pool behind my heart, flush down my spine, and fill my belly before pulsing out my limbs. I lose the edges of myself and am floating in this strange space that feels something like relief. The burning in my throat disappears. Only my jaw still hurts, from screaming as wide and loud as my mouth will let me.

"This might sound strange," Alan says after I tell him about my jaw, "but what if you just opened your mouth and pretended there's a rope coming out of it and the other end is in your body? Can we pull the rope out?"

Though I am alone, I still feel self-conscious about pulling a metaphorical rope out of my body at the suggestion of a man whose face I've never seen. But the fires in my mind are steaming now, doused in a strong rain. The forest floor is black and whatever trees are left hide in the mist, their bare, charred branches mere shadows in the fog. I open my mouth as wide as I can, my jaw clicking as I move it side to side. Hand over hand, I pull the rope out. Once I start pulling, it seems the rope is endless. I pull and pull and pull, imagining the frayed threads piling up on my desk in front of me. Hand over hand. Until I am empty. Until there is nothing left.

~~~~~~~~~~~~~~~~

The pitch and pattern of my screams became familiar. Before any sound shoots out of my mouth, my limbs burn as if the blood pulsing through my veins has turned to molten lead. Then I get lightheaded. Sound intensifies and my vision narrows. In public, I ball up my fists until the muscles in my forearms spasm in order to contain the buildup of energy. I hold it in until the moment I get home and I go to my bed and beat the mattress and strangle the pillows. Sometimes I fill up the bathtub, stick my face in the water, and scream. As I listen to the vibrations bounce off the porcelain, I think about keeping my head under and suffocating the scream, once and for all.

In between the screams I look around and see my world still chugs forward. I still need to get passport photos and vaccinated for malaria, yellow fever, Hepatitis A and B, Japanese encephalitis, and typhoid. I still need to find a dog walker that Buffy tolerates and convince my building to let me bring in a subletter. I still need to send *Chopped* a headshot, so I book an appointment with a photographer. On the day he arrives at my apartment, I spend most of the morning crying into a pillow. When the photographer sends me the edited files, all I see is pain. With yet another bucket of tears running down my cheeks, I whisper to the woman on the screen in front of me, "I'm so sorry you're sad." When the bucket finally empties, I blow my nose and send the photo off to the producers.

That's how the weeks pass. I cry. I scream. And in between I do the work. I call a clinic and make an appointment for vaccinations. I land a part time, remote job writing blog posts for a strength & fitness website. I find a loophole in my building's policies allowing for a one-time sublease in the event of occupational relocation, so I tell the board I am getting sent abroad for work and they approve a subletter. I make flashcards with endless flavor combinations and instructions for basic cooking techniques I haven't practiced since culinary school. Simmer fruit with vinegar and sugar for a quick gastrique. Cook venison to an internal temperature of 130 degrees and take soft caramel to 235 degrees. Pair strawberries with avocado, fennel, and mint. Tomatoes with peaches and Thai basil. Quick-cure fillets of fish under a pile of salt and sugar.

As the shoot date creeps closer, I convince friends to come over for dinner parties in which it is their job to scour the grocery store for four absurd ingredients, so I can do *Chopped* run-throughs. When they arrive at my apartment, they ask me where I've been and why my eyes are puffy. I lie. "Late spring allergies. Something in the air." This double life is not their burden, and I need their presence to divert my focus away from myself and onto the food. In the kitchen, with a timer and a problem to solve, the urge to hurt, scream, and destroy evaporates as it hits the searing-hot frying pan. I make pasta out of marshmallows, yellow peppers, and Pirate's Booty popcorn. Crab cakes turn into crab fried rice with pickled strawberries. Chicken thighs, Oreos, white-chocolate ice cream bars, and cauliflower become Oreo fried chicken with a spicy, white-chocolate cauliflower sauce. My friends don't just eat the food; they devour it and ask for more.

Still, I am convinced I will melt down on national television, crumble into a sobbing heap in the walk-in refrigerator or scream at a wheel of cheese from across the set. I schedule a session with Alan the day before *Chopped* films. He asks me to visualize myself standing in front of my first mystery basket. I close my eyes and imagine the *Chopped* kitchen. Four stations are lined up in a row, the judges on one end and the pantry on the other. Cameras dash all around. In front of me, there's an old-fashioned picnic basket filled with a mystery ingredient. I open it and peer inside. Right away, I freeze. The basket is filled with nothing but onions.

"I'm so sorry the puzzle was too hard."

All around me, the other chefs are dicing, sautéing, caramelizing. They have purpose, direction, a vision.

"I'm so sorry everything is so competitive."

I don't remember how onions taste.

"I'm so sorry it wasn't lighthearted and easy."

I pick up a knife. Grab an onion.

"I'm so sorry nothing is lighthearted and easy."

The knife slips.

"I'm so sorry everything is heavy and a struggle."

There is blood.

"I'm so sorry you didn't know what to do."

The set, my arms, my apron—nothing but red.

"I'm so sorry you're tired of struggling."

I don't belong here. I don't belong.

Alan stops and asks me to reset and try again. I close my eyes and cameras are still moving around the set. The judges whisper among themselves outside of my earshot. The kitchen seems cold, somehow, despite the roaring ovens and burners. The basket rests on my station, still filled with onions.

"I'm so sorry you couldn't use the problem to create a better outcome."

I open the mystery basket again and this time I pick a direction.

"I'm so sorry you couldn't see how to turn a difficult problem into a shining moment."

I take the onion. Dice it.

"I'm so sorry they set you up to fail."

My execution is sloppy and ugly.

"I'm so sorry they're laughing at you."

The judges snicker as they watch me struggle to put something on the plate.

"I'm so sorry they're enjoying your struggle."

The judges take a bite and see me for what I am: a fraud.

"I have a question," Alan says, taking a break from the statements.

"Okay," I say, blowing my nose into squares of toilet paper and sniffing into the phone. I don't even know if I should bother showing up to the shoot if I can't even visualize myself chopping an onion without hitting an artery.

Alan asks, with total seriousness, "In this visualization, are the judges able to feel the love in your food? Can you ask the judges if they can feel the love?"

I sigh into the phone.

As if love is enough to counter years of actual kitchen experience, not bullshit cupcake baking in a claustrophobic basement. Of course they can't feel the love.

I purse my lips, clamp my jaw, and close my eyes, entertaining the question only because I'm already here, paying for this. I may as well not fight it and just do what the man says. The judges sit across from me in my mind's eye, each one a faceless blob, illuminated in their own little spotlight.

I ask them, *"Can you feel the love?"* and wait for the answer. One shrugs. Another backs away and dissolves into the darkness. One shakes its formless head.

"No, Alan. They can't." I drop my own head in shame. Even in my fantasies I can't deliver.

"Okay, let's do some compassion on that. Take a big breath and feel into your solar plexus, and when we go through the statements this time I want you to pour love into the food. As much as you can. See it filling the plate. Now repeat after me: I'm so sorry they couldn't receive the love."

I take two onions and throw them into the food processor.

"I'm so sorry they couldn't taste the love."

A hot pan. A splash of oil. A sizzle.

"I'm so sorry their critical minds got in the way."

I run to the refrigerator. The pantry. Handfuls of herbs and cream and stock.

"I'm so sorry they weren't capable of experiencing what you gave them."

A pot bubbles over and another chef slams down a plate.

"I'm so sorry they were injured themselves and couldn't fully receive your love."

I arrange the dishes. Ladle the soup.

"I'm so sorry they broke your heart."

I pour all I am into the bowl.

Alan and I work together for two hours, eventually managing to get me through a full visualization of the appetizer, entrée, and dessert rounds that avoids the chopping block each time. A subtle confidence prickles at me and I feel into the sensation of winning, of redeeming myself from all of my perceived failures—balking on the diving board in college, losing my twenties to dark depression, a lemon of a business partnership. For the first time, I think I can make it through filming without deteriorating into tears.

But that night, as I settle into my flashcards, a burst of rage emerges that is so strong and deep I punch my thighs until they are splattered with crimson speckles. I hit them until all the energy is out of me, until my skin is numb. Then I thank my legs for taking a beating and return to the information on the flashcards in front of me: Scallops in the shell have a muscle that must be removed. Nettles need to be blanched in order to erase the sting. Black pepper enhances the sweetness of plums.

10

I lay awake all night, debating whether to show up for the *Chopped* 5 a.m. call time. I only decide to go after realizing how many people I would piss off if I didn't show up.

I am the first to arrive at the coffee shop across from the studio where all the *Chopped* contestants are supposed to meet. I order a drink just to have something to hold onto. My stomach is already in knots, and the coffee only churns it more.

One by one the other contestants arrive: Doug, a tall, gentle thirtysomething who is the head chef at a museum in Baltimore; Jenny, a Chinese-American prodigy who pivoted to culinary arts after becoming the youngest candidate in history at Columbia Business School; and Arnaud, a tight-lipped Frenchman with more cooking experience than the rest of us combined. As the three of them compare résumés, I hug my coffee cup. It's like I brought a spoon to knife fight, but it's too late to turn back.

Four *Chopped* producers, one for each of us, arrive at the coffee shop and walk us to the studio across the street. I recognize my producer, Maya, from my on-camera casting interview. I relax a little when she re-introduces herself, glad to have a familiar face around.

"I told you that you had a decent shot," she says as we pass through security.

"I almost didn't show up," I say, shaking as I hand her all my personal belongings. Anything that gives contestants an edge or connects them to the outside world—phones, notebooks, kitchen tools—gets locked up for the day.

"Whatever is going to happen is going to happen," Maya says. "Try to have some fun with it."

I swallow a mouthful of bile as Maya leads me to the *Chopped* kitchen, a sprawling television set with a pantry on one end, a judging table on the other, and four cooking stations in between. I am assigned cooking station number one, the farthest from the judges but closest to the pantry. Doug is next to me, followed by Arnaud and Jenny.

The four of us are given an extensive tour of the kitchen and taught how to use the equipment. We turn on the stove, check the oven, and browse the pantry, taking mental notes of where everything is located. By design, there is only one of everything in the kitchen—one ice-cream maker, one fryer, one bunch of parsley. If you need something someone else is using, you better hope they're nice enough to share.

We are all mic'd up, given a *Chopped* chef's jacket, and escorted to the sequester room, where we wait until filming begins. The room looks like a working kitchen, but none of the appliances are hooked up. The four of us stare at each other, fidget, and make awkward jokes. A production assistant, whose only job is to keep eyeballs on the contestants, sits on a chair a few feet away.

"You guys are lucky," the PA says. "There's almost always one jerk in the group who talks shit before anyone gets to show what they can do. None of you seem like assholes."

~~~~~~~~~~

As we line up to march out to the kitchen for the first round, Maya gives me a pep talk.

"You're going to walk out there with confidence and smile for the camera. I need big enthusiasm. Got it?"

I nod, pacing. All the tension is transforming into frenetic energy I cannot contain, the nodules in my arms throbbing. I hear the *Chopped* host, Ted Allen, introduce me on set.

"You got this," Maya says. "Go!"

I plaster a fake smile on my face and walk into the *Chopped* kitchen. I recognize two of the three judges from other *Chopped* episodes: pastry chef Zac Young and Indian-born, Nashville-nurtured chef Maneet Chauhan. The third judge is Katrina Markoff, a chocolatier brought in to guest-judge our chocolate-themed episode. Cameramen roam about, capturing footage of me from all angles as I walk to my station. I chew the skin off my lip while the other three chefs are introduced, staring at the mystery basket in front of me.

When we are instructed to open the first mystery basket in the *Chopped* kitchen, I find pomegranate seeds, white chocolate-covered caviar, chocolate olive oil, and a dozen wiggling soft-shell crabs staring back at me. The starting buzzer rings and I panic. I've never worked with soft-shell crabs. I know they need to be cleaned, but I have no idea how to clean them. I do the only thing I can think of and run to the refrigerator, grab an onion, and say, "I make goddamned cupcakes for a living. This is fucking ridiculous."

I hear the producers giggle and feel the stare of half a dozen cameras on me. I dice the onion and curse myself for showing up this morning, any confidence I gained during my session with Alan melted away. Now, faced with a pile of crabs trying to escape their fate, I decide my only job is to fight back tears.

"Take the scissors and cut off its face." Chef Doug leans over from the station next to me and holds a limp crab over my cutting board. "Then pull out the sac and cut out the gills. I'm from Baltimore. We do this all the time."

I watch him plow through his basket of crabs in a matter of seconds, dumbstruck by both his speed and generosity. Doug is my competition. And yet he may have just saved me. Over the next ten minutes, I mutilate the basket of crabs, burn a pan full of chocolate olive oil, forget every knife skill I've ever learned, and just when I get my shit together long enough to take a breath, I knock one of my four deep-fried, breadcrumb, and paprika-crusted crabs onto the floor.

Lightning speed comes to a halt and for a moment I consider picking up the crab. I know I can't serve the fallen crustacean, but I also need to present four complete plates—three for the judges and one for the film crew for a beauty shot. Now I'm down a crab. Despite the run-throughs, studying, and hours of work I put in with Alan last night, going home seems inevitable after this round. I am embarrassed to admit I thought I could get through this experience with a smidgen of grace, and that the visualizations would translate into a positive outcome. I was right to be skeptical of Alan's process and claims. Clearly, it doesn't work. I have the crab to prove it.

I decide I don't want to be responsible for someone's twisted ankle on top of culinary embarrassment, so I reach down to the floor to pick up the poor crab and hear the supervising producer bellow through the clangs of pots and pans:

"Leave it!" A cameraman comes out of nowhere, crouches on the floor, and gets a close-up of my crab. I can already see how this will be edited for television. The camera will zoom in on my crab, dramatic "DUN DUNNNN" notes alerting viewers that a *Chopped* tragedy has occurred. I know that my inability to control my crabs is going to be part of the episode teaser. My clumsiness will be immortalized, perhaps even syndicated. Hell, this could end up on Netflix.

"How you doing, chef?" Doug yells out to me from his station, snapping me out of my stupor. I look at Doug, who is wildly whisking something on the stove with an encouraging grin. I shrug, take a dramatic breath. I don't have time to clean and bread another crab, so I grab one from the basket and drop it naked into the deep fryer. There is still some time on the clock. I can at least get something on all four plates.

I throw together a haphazard presentation of deep-fried soft-shell crab served with a white-chocolate pomegranate sauce, shaved brussels sprouts, and a chocolate olive oil vinaigrette. I make a crack to the judges about how one of them got the "light" version. I get a laugh, but the judges still rip apart my dish for a half hour, complimenting only the white-chocolate pomegranate sauce. They grill me about the crab and pin Doug into a corner by asking him how he's going to feel if I make it through the round and he doesn't. As the classiest person in the room, he responds, "Good for her."

We break for the judges' deliberation and I burst into tears, humiliated by my performance. Maya pulls me aside. She tells me I need to relax because either my day will be over in five minutes or I have to do this all over again. She gives me a tissue to wipe my eyes and I am sent back to the judges.

The eliminated dish sits under a silver cloche on the corner of the table, waiting to be revealed. We all know Doug and Arnaud are safe. The judges liked their dishes, and neither one of them had technical problems. Jenny's crab was a touch raw in the middle, but the judges fawned over her flavors. Between floor crab and raw crab, I figure she's got the edge.

Ted lifts the cloche and reveals the chopped dish—Jenny's. I am flooded with equal amounts of exhilaration and terror. On the one hand, I made it to the second round. On the other, I have to go through this hell again, and I can't entirely be sure if that's better.

"You dodged a bullet," Maneet says to me, without an ounce of levity. "Step it up."

More familiar with the kitchen and the feeling of performing under pressure, I settle down in the next round and channel the stress into the next mystery basket. I get to work on smoked pork shanks, a chocolate crepe cake, purple spinach, and chocolate whiskey. I shred the pork off the bones and smother it in a sauce made from the chocolate crepe cake and half the spice pantry. It's like an open bottle of Memphis barbecue sauce fell into a simmering pot of Mexican *mole negro*, creating a happy accident of sweet, savory tang that pairs perfectly with the smoky pork. I wilt the spinach with a splash of whiskey to cut the richness and serve it over a potato puree. I undercook the potatoes and nearly tank the whole dish, but it's not as bad as Arnaud, who gets chopped after attempting to turn the pork into a chocolate sausage that looks like, unfortunately, a literal pile of shit.

Then there are two.

Doug and I face off over the dessert round and, for the first time all day, I feel like maybe I can win this. After all, I make cupcakes for a living. The one time it comes in handy. Doug is frantic at his station, but he's too far away for me to know what's going right or wrong. It's only when we get back to the sequester room that he tells me he spent thirty minutes trying, and failing, to toast bread for a dessert panini. When his soggy sandwich appears on the chopping block, I feel the heat of the cameras zoom in on me.

I won.

I don't breathe. I don't blink. I am a mass of confused, elated, dumbstruck joy. The floor falls away and I am whisked off for a two-hour interview to relive the day. Maya asks me questions and it's like she's speaking to me through water. Her voice swirls around me and I internalize what she's saying just enough to talk, but my mind is elsewhere, fixated on this high.

This is new.

It feels almost chemical, like the buildup of stress transformed into an instant rush of intoxicating serotonin and dopamine. I know this euphoria is circumstantial, that it's one end of a bell curve that will inevitably right its way back to center when the television lights turn off. But I've never wandered near this side of the bell curve before, and I am fascinated by it. Until now, I believed the endgame of antidepressant withdrawal was simply that I would no longer teeter on the edge of collapse, but that I would still be left a person who, by nature, trends toward melancholy. Now, soaked in euphoria and splattered with chocolaty remnants of culinary war, I realize how much unexplored space lies on the bright side of the curve. I won't live in this state of bliss forever. Maybe I can live near it. Or even within its city limits. At the very least, maybe I can pop over for a visit now and then.

By the time I get home it is nearly midnight and I am still wired, pumped full of adrenaline. I stand up. I sit down. I walk from my desk to the kitchen to the bedroom and turn in wild circles and jump up and down and shake the electricity from my body. I email Alan with the news, which technically breeches the contract I signed with Food Network. I know he won't violate our confidentiality agreement, and he has to be told our work paid off. My eyes fill with tears as I type. Tears of relief.

I pull out my watercolors and fumble through my knife roll for my favorite, a Wusthof seven-inch santoku I've used for eight years. The knife is heavy in my hand, still razor-sharp despite the day of use. It is a workhorse, not flashy or high-end, made of German steel strong enough to cut through bone and delicate enough to mince herbs without bruising their tender leaves. It's been with me since culinary school, guided me through Manhattan kitchens, helped me open a bakery, and led me to not just a *Chopped* win, but a breakthrough.

For all these years, there was always a way to dig a little deeper into depression, to let my body and mind sink a little more into the darkness and root around for a place to sleep, never coming up for light. Bright, shiny mornings were for other people, whose bodies and minds churned out adrenaline and joy and pleasure. Today, with this knife, my world turned from flat to round, the edge of the horizon not fading to nothing, but revealing a whole other side of the emotional spectrum I never knew existed within me. I want to immortalize it, to fill it with this feeling so I remember what is possible.

I place the knife on top of a clean sheet of paper and trace its edges. I lift it from the paper and fill in its details, measuring out the precise distance between each of the handle's three studs. I take a pencil-thin brush and line the blade's outline with water, then use a pipette to flush the blade. The droplets merge together in perfect form, filling in the flat outline of the knife into three dimensions. I drip single beads of magenta, yellow, fuchsia, and orange paint into the shallow pool of water held in tight by tensile edges.

Drip, drip, drip.

I think back to the raindrops and the sting of their edges, the first sign of awakening after a fifteen-year hibernation. It was as if my body was covered in a layer of cellophane that raindrops could never penetrate. On that spring night the cellophane lifted and suddenly I could feel the rain. I stood on the sidewalk and watched the droplets cascade from my shoulders to my fingers, creating little rivers and waterfalls.

Now, I begin to remember all of the times when I simply just got wet, memories that had long ago fallen out of my head.

Drip, drip, drip.

I remember watching a thunderstorm in rural North Carolina with my first New York City boyfriend, and how the midday sky turned black as night over the cornfields. I remember walking home to my college dorm through a rainstorm after a long night of studying for my freshman year oceanography course. The smell of rain on red maple trees was mustier than the sweet crispness of Nevada's rain on dust. I remember when my mother told me about her breast cancer diagnosis, just a year or so after my father passed.

"I'm not dying," she told me matter-of-factly. "I have way too much left to do."

Drip, drip, drip.

I remember sitting in a parking lot in my father's car and listening to the rain patter on the sunroof in the months after he died. I remember the thunderstorm from the night he died, too. Lightning snaked across Washoe Valley and a burst of rain came as quickly as it went, cooling the sweltering July earth.

Drip, drip, drip.

I remember the gray curls of the Naples taxi driver bouncing as he sped over potholes, determined to get my mother and me to the airport before the first of four flights left to take us home to my comatose father. The individual cobblestones on the street glistened in the moonlight, newly wet from an evening storm.

Drip, drip, drip.

Explosions of magenta and yellow and fuchsia and orange swirl together on the page creating galaxies of color swirling into the knife's blade. The paint envelops each molecule of water until the santoku-shaped puddle is fat with color and I wonder when the bubble will burst and if I've added too much color and what this will look like in the morning. I can't stop the energy and I won't stop the vibrance or the beauty so I paint and paint and paint.

Drip, drip, drip.

Each droplet sings.

I float through Manhattan for twenty-four hours before my victorious haze dissipates into the sticky summer heat, replaced by a whiplash of paranoia that engulfs me with unexpected force. I am waiting for the uptown 6 train at Union Square when I read the news of the first ever ISIS attack in Malaysia, the latest in a string of terrorist attacks making headlines all over the globe.

I push the incident out of my mind as the downtown subway train comes barreling through the station with a screech that seems to slice open my eardrums. I cover my ears with my hands like a child. I do not lower my arms until the train pulls away and takes the shriek of metal on metal with it. This city feels louder now than ever before, a crushing vortex of energy I cannot turn down. In a few hours this platform will be stuffed with thousands of people, each one praying for the train's precious wind offering a few seconds of relief from the stifling heat. I will not be here, packed into the station shoulder to sweaty shoulder. I don't take the train at rush hour anymore. I don't go to Times Square or the Empire State Building either. It is all too loud. Too busy. Too dangerous.

I try to pull my mind from the fear of impending terrorism and focus on the details of my new world, a world without antidepressants for ninety-nine days. I scan the few people around me and see the pores on their faces and the color gradients in each strand of their hair. White headphone cords hang limp against their skin, and the colors of each sweat-stained T-shirt speckle the gray subway station like drops of paint dried on a garage floor. The world has settled into focus, true focus, and I feel like I've been skinned. Not only have the edges sharpened and the colors brightened, but all that is ugly has magnified too. I notice every ten-foot pile of garbage, every swatch of graffiti marring the walls, every addict picking scabs off his shins. I am terrified of the world around me. Terrified of debilitating illness and war and death, of broken bones and hearts and promises.

I get off all this medication and this is what I wake up to? It's dirty and dangerous and the joy is not as strong as the despair and it all ends in piles of trash and sadness, and how is life worth living when one terrible person can walk into an airport and kill the good in dozens? Why bother living when everything beautiful is so easily destroyed?

I try to feel into the elation of winning *Chopped* and the peace of painting deep into the night. But withdrawal takes me so far up and then crashes me back down, reminding me that existence hurts much more than it ever did before, when the pills allowed me to feel only just enough.

Even the heat hurts. I am an ant caught in tar. The intensity wraps around me, and I stand with my feet wide and my arms floating a few inches away from my torso, feeling the beads of sweat rolling down my skin and changing course with each tender lump on my limbs. The biopsy results still haven't come in, so I jump from cancerous scenario to cancerous scenario, creating opposing worlds in my head. One is full of IVs and hospitals and medical bills. In another, I just let go. I let the cancer take me. I don't go to doctors. I don't go to chemotherapy. I don't fight. I welcome the inevitability of imminent death and am grateful to leave, gone before I have a chance to witness the spectacular implosion of the human race.

I feel the push of air from an oncoming train. It's not my train, but for a few seconds I have a break from the heat. I breathe in and feel the wet air fill my lungs and, for an instant, I am alive and I am glad to be alive and maybe this too will pass. The train passes and my glimmer of light goes with it as the heat settles on my body, sending my thoughts back to the lumps on my arms and how it would feel to just let them fester until they take me away. I am jolted out of my daydream by the sound of a plastic stroller hitting the walls of the subway stairwell behind me. A distinct chill comes through my body and, without turning around, I know the energy in the station has shifted. I check the screen hanging from the ceiling of the subway. My local train is eight minutes away. The express will be here in three minutes.

I look over my shoulder toward the continuing commotion. A family of five huddles close together on the platform, the father standing behind the stroller. From a distance, they seem like a family visiting New York City, out to see the sites and enjoy the city. But up close, standing next to them, something is off. A girl, perhaps six years old and clearly too large for the stroller, tucks into its canvas sling and stares straight ahead. She is dressed in pink leggings and a white-and-pink floral shirt, identical to her two sisters who are anywhere from ten to fourteen years old. All three of them have long, black hair, pulled into limp ponytails at the nape of their necks. Their mother stands in ill-fitting clothes—baggy jeans, a long-sleeved shirt—and has the same ponytail as her daughters. She has a large I Heart NY canvas bag slung over her shoulder and looks away from her husband, who stands with a camera around his neck that is at least two decades old, but oddly seems to be unused. He wears brand-new blue jeans still creased from their package, a souvenir New York City T-shirt, and a distinct beard, long and unkempt with a deliberate lack of mustache, a style distinct to both Brooklyn hipsters and the ultra-conservative jihadists I've seen on the news.

The family does not speak. They move like robots and do not make eye contact with each other or anyone else. They seem unclear in where they are going, but don't consult a map or ask for directions. The children don't look around or fiddle with their hair or complain about the heat. The man grips the handles of the stroller so tight his knuckles are white. Maybe they are refugees. Maybe they are scared. Maybe I am a piece of shit for even thinking this way, but every fiber in my body is lighting up and telling me something about this situation is off, so I back away from the family as a train pulls into the station and I get on it because part of me is terrified and part of me is ashamed, and I don't know what is right and I will never know what is right. All I know is I am scared.

I get home and slump down at my computer and start to Google the influence of extremist groups in Malaysia. A counterterrorism website tells me that, in January, Malaysian ISIS fighters in Syria were featured in a video calling for "lone wolf" attacks in their home countries. It also says Malaysian police have arrested more than one hundred people for ISIS-related activities and that the ISIS suicide bomber who killed four people at a Starbucks in Jakarta was arrested in Kuala Lumpur.

I should learn some self-defense. Or at least how to throw a punch.

I open a new tab on my browser and search for self-defense gyms within walking distance of my apartment. It doesn't take long before I remember I live in New York City; throwing a punch couldn't save anyone in the Twin Towers.

Aren't we due for another terrorist attack?

I think about Times Square, all the subway rides, baseball games, and Thanksgiving Day parades filled with so many people in one space. And because I'm completely fucked in the head, the fact that a successful attack hasn't happened in this city since 9/11 prompts a thought, aimed at no terrorist group in particular:

You're really bad at your job. I would be a better terrorist than you.

At the conclusion of this horrific notion I slam my computer shut and push back from my desk. Maybe I need to forget this whole thing. Forget Remote Year. Forget New York City. Just move to a cabin in the middle of Idaho, with nothing but the rustle of grass and a few cows to keep me company.

Then again, Idaho couldn't save Hemingway.

But at least in Idaho I could breathe, knowing I was far away from the targets of ISIS and Boko Haram. They're everywhere now, it seems. They might be everywhere I'm going, too.

I shift my gaze to the painted knife lying next to my computer, fat droplets now dried flat. I run my fingers over the blade and feel the warped paper saturated with color. There is a distinct change in texture at the knife's edge where the color begins, swirls of wet paint now settled into what looks like a technicolor wave crashing onto an otherworldly shore. On one side of the blade, near the handle, a marigold tide engulfs coral sand. But near the tip, the wave seems to pull away, leading to a calm magenta sea. I can't ignore the symbol in the accidental art, how the blade churns in brilliant color but ultimately stills.

Alan's voice flows through my mind. *I'm so sorry you can't trust the ground you walk on.*

"I'm so sorry you can't trust the ground you walk on," I whisper, and let the glimmer of relief from the words flow through me.

11

I blink and I am in Reno. The desert night envelops me as the plane lands, and when I step outside of the airport I stop and let the quiet wash through me. Everything I know is gone.

New York. My bakery. My business partner. My apartment. My home. My friends. My old body and mind and self. Gone. Abandoned. And Buffy, my little Demon Dog. She's with Dolores. They're slow and old and happy together, and when I land in Reno I get an email from Dolores: "Buffy and I are still as adorable as ever. We are so lucky and glad you brought us together. She makes my heart sing."

Boiling-hot grief steams inside me, but the midnight Nevada air is crisp and cools me from the outside in. I look up to the darkness and find the light. I can't remember the last time I saw stars so bright against a pitch-black night. The moon hangs above me with the sort of obvious presence found only in nursery rhymes and cartoons. I look deep into its highlights and shadows and a face appears: the Man in the Moon. Of course, I know about the Man in the Moon, but I've never been able see him. More than once, I've stood with friends as they tried to point out the craters creating the illusion of a face gazing upon Earth with a look of surprise and a touch of pity.

"See the man? See the moon?" they asked.

I always shook my head. For the life of me, I could not see the damn man in the damn moon. But here he is, found in the same patchy, dark spots I'd examined so many times before, so plain and obvious I cannot comprehend how I missed him for all these years.

Edges, I suppose.

My mother pulls up to the curb and I load my single suitcase into the car before falling into her arms. She drives us home and I press my cheek against the window, watching the cosmos turn around me.

I have twenty-seven days in Reno. Twenty-seven days to right myself, screw my head on straight, get a diagnosis on the lumps in my arms, and pack a life into a suitcase and two backpacks. I need to go to the safety-deposit box and dig out my worn yellow-fever card. I need vacuum-seal packing bags and a toiletry set, a power strip for my electronics and extra batteries, a water purifier and a packet of anti-diarrhea medication just in case the water purifier fails. I need a bathing suit for Thailand in October and a heavy jacket for Prague in January. I need earplugs. Sunglasses. An over-the-shoulder bag with a strap that can't be slashed with a pocketknife. Condoms. Do I need condoms? I stuff one in my purse just in case. Along with a spork.

With all the vaccines for mosquito-borne illness I wonder if I need a mosquito net, too. So I buy one. According to the internet, DEET is more effective than citronella, so I buy four bottles off Amazon in a panic. The bottles sit on the ping-pong table in my mother's basement, along with a year's worth of stuff. It is all too much space.

I am too much space.

The nodules in my arms throb as I wonder how all of this space will pack into a suitcase, how it will survive a trek across the world, if any of this is even worth it. There is no joy strewn across the ping-pong table, only obligation born out of a desperate need to get away, to make a different choice, to do something—anything—differently. That's the honest, ugly truth. I know people who would salivate over this opportunity, people who go blind with rage during hour-long commutes between a house filled with screaming kids and a job filled with screaming managers. I know this isn't the sort of opportunity you get twice, that it's either take it and run or leave it and regret. I know I should be grateful.

But fuck gratitude. Gratitude is the bow we tie around our brand of shit to convince ourselves our particular pile of shit is a pretty pile of shit.

I wrap my arms around myself, but my limbs are so tender I pull away at my own touch. How can I be grateful for this? Gratitude is no match for grief, loss, the untrodden path of phenomenal change. I am mourning the loss of my life, my self. I know only the woman—the girl—who for fifteen years stood stoic and anesthetized, waiting to dissolve into nothing. I do not know this woman, this sniffling, screaming, scared woman hoarding an arsenal of mosquito repellants. I do not understand her. I don't know what she wants. I don't know what she believes and I don't know what she needs. I don't know how to get to know her, how to see her, how to live with her. All I know is there is no going back, not to that girl or to New York. Someone else is living in my home. Someone else is walking my dog. Someone else is running my business. That life doesn't belong to me anymore. All that belongs to me is piled on this ping-pong table.

I'm so sorry you can't go back to before you were broken.

My mother comes shuffling down the stairs in her fuzzy robe and slippers, almonds piled in her hand.

"How you doing, sweetheart?"

I turn around to face her, the circles under my eyes dark and swollen and wet. I hold out my arms, lumpy and bruised.

"My legs look like this too," I tell her. Then I collapse onto her shoulder and sob.

———————

The next day, my mother convinces me to take a mosaic art class with her. To move the energy. To do something creative. To focus on something I can touch. A rare summer rain pounds on the car as we drive, covering the windows in glittery droplets blurring the outside world and encasing my mother and me into our own.

"Are you any better today, honey?" my mother asks.

"What?" I say, snapping out of my nervous mental loop. I look around and realize we are parked, but we are early. The art studio doors are locked. My mother turns off the car and we wait.

"No," I say in a low voice, shaking my head.

"I'm so sorry, sweetheart."

My mother takes my hand, holds it. The rain patters all around us.

"This just doesn't seem worth it," I say after a moment of silence.

"What's not worth it?" my mother asks.

"*This.*" I break our handhold and gesture around the car, as if it encased all the space in the world. "All of this. Seriously, what's the point? What was the point of getting off the antidepressants when all it did was illuminate how shitty people are, and how much ugliness there is? At least on the drugs, none of it mattered. Dead. Alive. Whatever. It all felt more or less the same. It all seemed better that way."

"No. *No.*" My mother raises her voice. "It was *not* better. You were scaring the hell out of me. The last time I came to New York you couldn't get off the couch. And then—I'll never forget it—you were home from New York and you crawled into bed with me and all the life in your eyes was gone." My mother closes her eyes and grips the steering wheel. "I knew you were wrong about being 'born broken.' I knew because I raised you. I knew that person. I knew that heart. You were always intense. But so what? I'm intense. Your father was intense. Of course you were going to be intense."

"But that's what I can't figure out. What part of this is me and what part is withdrawal? Am I still even in withdrawal? Or is this just the same, old depression talking? Or is it not withdrawal or depression or dad's bullshit and it's just a fucking blind spot in my personality?"

"I don't know, honey. All I can tell you is who you were as a kid, before all of this. You laughed. You were curious. You were sensitive and tough at the same time. Then it stopped. Your father died and you started taking the antidepressants and all that made you *you* just stopped."

My mother reaches into her pocket, pulls out a wadded-up tissue, and blows her nose. She is crying now. I am too.

"I did the best I could," she says, sniffling and refolding the tissue. My mother grabs my hand again. "You were totally shut down. You wouldn't talk to me. That child psychologist wouldn't talk to me. She just called me one day and said she couldn't discuss details with me, but that I was wasting my money on therapy, and prescription medication was the next step. Kathy agreed. Your father wasn't here. You weren't eating. I didn't know what else to do."

My mother looks at me and seems to transform into an old woman. I see every worry line, wrinkle, and burden she's carried all these years. I want to go back in time and be a better daughter. I want to hug her, comfort her, take the pain away from her.

"I don't blame you for any of this. You have to know that," I tell her. And it's true.

"I did the best I could with the information I had at the time," she says. "If I had known what I know now, if I could have seen how hard it's been for you to get off them . . . "

I interrupt. "Honestly we probably would have made the same choice. It was a different time. No one could have predicted this."

"Maybe."

The art studio's doors are open now. We watch a few people shake off the rain and enter the building.

"You don't have to go right now if you don't want to," my mother says.

"To the art class or on Remote Year?"

"Well, either. But I meant Remote Year. If you're not ready, you could change your flight. Meet the group in Europe. You can stay here as long as you want."

"Staying in Reno isn't the answer."

We both go quiet.

"Did you think the Prozac made a difference for dad?" I ask.

My mother shrugs. "I don't know, maybe. He still threw his epic tantrums. Maybe they were less frequent. What I remember him saying was he didn't like how the Prozac affected his mind. He said it made him slow, like he was trying to think through soup. And you know how quick his mind was."

"Why did you put up with him for so long?"

"It was kind of all I knew. My father could be mean. All the men in my family were verbal abusers. And your father's father, he treated Grandma like your father treated me. Your father never hit me. I guess on some level I thought that was enough. I professed to be a feminist, but that was all talk. Underneath, I didn't know how to be a feminist."

"What about when he knocked you around in the boat when you found out you were pregnant?"

My mother pauses, takes a breath. "I didn't understand that he was trying to make me miscarry. I don't think I was able to understand it. My mind wouldn't allow me to. It sounds odd, but at the time I was just mad about how rough he was being with my father's boat and how he didn't care about me being tossed around.

"He wasn't all bad. He wasn't a total monster. Once, he even said to me, from the bottom of his heart, 'Can you ever forgive me for all the things I've done to you?'"

I shake my head. "That's not enough."

"No. But about a couple of years before he died, I finally found the courage to stand up to him. He was throwing one of his fits and I said, 'Shape up or we're leaving. Brooke and I can't live like this.' He walked over to me, bent over, and got an inch from my face. He was so much bigger than me. I expected him to blow like he had so many times before. Instead he said, cool as a cucumber, 'And you shouldn't have to.' Everything was different from that moment on."

"What shifted?" I ask, trying to understand how to flip the switch.

"I think in some ways, I had to learn to stand up for myself. To find my own voice and say enough is enough. Your father didn't believe in divorce. Maybe the threat scared him straight. Maybe it was the cancer messing with his brain, I don't know. He was wonderful in those last years. He rode his motorcycle a lot, which he loved. He volunteered at an at-risk middle school. He was a Big Brother. We laughed. They were the best years of our marriage. For the first time, he seemed at peace."

Through the art studio's windows, we can see the instructor handing out supplies. Neither one of us makes a move to get out of the car. I don't know what to say or where to begin untangling the thread of responsibility. It's why I don't hold an ounce of resentment toward my mother for putting me on antidepressants. The story began long before that moment, before I was born, before she was born.

"I'm so proud of you," my mother says.

I raise an eyebrow, dumbfounded. "Why?"

"Because you're not boring. It's always been an adventure with you. You forge your own path and now you're facing all the things you need to fix in your life. You're doing it at thirty. Most people don't sort themselves out until they're my age, if they ever do it at all. And that's the whole point of being human, of being *here*."

"I'd kill for a little less adventure and a little more obliviousness."

"That's never been who you are. You were never typical. There was one time when you were a toddler, and I came into the room and found you standing, *standing* on your rocking horse and rocking like crazy with a big smile on your face. Or when you were thirteen and you went to Australia all by yourself with that foreign-exchange program. Other parents thought we were out of our minds for letting you go. But you were with a reputable organization and I knew you could handle it. I also know you can handle this. You've handled everything that's come at you so far. I always trust you to handle it. Moving to New York by yourself. Opening the bakery. *Chopped.*"

"I had help with all of those things."

"Everyone has help," my mother says. "We don't do anything in this world alone. For God's sake, if I had any sort of intuition anything was going to happen to you on Remote Year, I wouldn't let you go. People keep asking me how I can let you travel all around the world when ISIS is blowing people up, but I know you're going to be safe. I'm solid on that."

I look at her, nod. The old woman I saw before me disappears and all I see is my mother's beautiful, glowing face. In that moment, I choose to believe her. I choose to believe in my heart that I will be okay, even if my mind is telling me otherwise.

We arrive late to the art class, the other students already tending to long tables filled with every color and texture of mosaic tiles. The instructor gives my mother and me each a board and a stapled packet of directions and the history of mosaic art. My mother studies the packet and gravitates toward gold, sienna clay, and sage-green tiles. I toss the packet aside, wait for the tiles to get picked over. When the table clears I take anything black and red and pile the tiles in front of me. Some are shiny, others are matte with swirls of gold. All have edges that scratch. I don't sketch an outline. I don't work off a photo. I just begin to glue red shards of tesserae onto the base, with no particular plan, until a shape begins to form. I end up with something resembling a geometric, blood-red money bag, stuffed full and cinched at the top with twine.

"What is it?" my mother asks, her Tuscan landscape morphing into view.

"I don't know. A sack of some sort?" I say, propping the board upright to get a better look.

"Whatever it is, it's very you—all that intensity with the black and red."

"This sounds so stupid when I say it out loud, but I feel like this is my depression. It's all stuffed into this bag-thing that comes with me wherever I go." I start gluing black tiles around the red bag, pronouncing the edges of a part of my life I would rather forget.

My mother is still looking over my shoulder, contemplating.

"Maybe it is the depression," she says, "but, look, it's contained within the bag. You don't have to take it with you. Maybe you leave it here, in the mosaic. You move forward without it."

My mother rubs my back and returns to her piece. I finish the black background, fill in the big gaps with mirror shards, and flood the spaces in between the tiles with grout. Part of me wants to throw this thing in the dumpster on my way out. Another part wants to mount it on the wall like a plaque acknowledging the completion of a grueling task.

The instructor comes by and gazes at my mother's work. She compliments her color selection, the delicate placement of her tesserae, and how her Tuscan hills gently rise. When the instructor gets to me, she cocks her head and narrows her eyes.

"Well that's different!" she says, "What is it? A cat? I see a cat."

I hold up the mosaic, look back to the instructor, nod my head.

"You're very perceptive," I tell her. "It's just a standard house cat. Meow."

12

Eleven bombs explode across Thailand, targeting tourism hotspots. Four people killed. Thirty-six injured. No terrorist organization takes responsibility.

Thailand is our second destination on the Remote Year itinerary. After five weeks in Kuala Lumpur, we are to spend the next five weeks on Koh Phangan, an island sixty miles off the mainland. I Google the island and see that the beaches are milky-white, the oceans turquoise and opaline with palms framing the coast. I wonder what lies out of the frame, what lurks in the corners of the island deemed too unsightly to photograph. There is darkness there, there has to be. Where there is light there is dark, the frayed cords of human experience braided in between. The question I keep asking myself: *Is it worth it?*

A fit of rage builds up in me in an instant and before I know it my stomach is tight and my vision goes red and my fists hit my thighs and I scream until my voice goes hoarse and my mother's dog, Luigi, darts out of the room.

I take myself down into my bedroom. Curl into a ball, hit the pillows, scream into the comforter.

Somewhere deep within my mind, a clear and calm thought: *Let it out.*

I hit, I shake, I wail for ten minutes, twenty minutes, an hour.

I finally close my eyes and the heaving slows and I try to rest, to reset. But as I lose my edges in the embrace of slumber I hear something in the distance—a rumbling, sporadic vroom. Coming closer. Getting louder. A chorus of leaf blowers.

The gardeners descend on the house like maggots on a fresh carcass, whirring their hell machines in nauseating cacophony. Front yard, back yard, side yard—the sound bores so deep into my body that my stomach churns and I dry heave foamy drops of bile onto the bedspread. I try to roll over, sit up, get away from the noise, but it's like the force of the leaf blowers skewers me to the bed, taking a hold of my nervous system. I wrap a pillow around my head and pin it against my ears, cinching myself into a tighter and tighter ball and begging for peace. But it doesn't stop for five minutes, ten minutes, twenty. I don't know how long it continues. I want to go into the back yard and snatch the leaf blowers from the men's soiled hands and heave the machine at their heads and beat them with it until all that is left is brain matter and grass just waiting to be raked up.

I think of my father and all the noise he made in the garage, revving his motorcycle at 7:00 a.m. on a Sunday. I think of how he yelled "son of a bitch!" and slammed an oil pan onto the cement floor. I think of how the neighbors complained and how he'd stomp out into the driveway and retort "it's my goddamn house!" and then return to changing lightbulbs or vacuuming the garage floor.

I think of him. He would have stormed out the back door and told the gardeners to use a goddamn rake or get off his lawn. I yearn for his confidence, his ego. His I-don't-give-a-shit-what-you-or-anyone-else-thinks attitude that gave him the freedom and space to blow and demand the world bow to him no matter who was around to see it. I want to find him in myself. And to never be like him.

I call Alan for an emergency session. He is exuberant and asks if I'm looking forward to leaving. Instead of matching his enthusiasm I go on a ten-minute cry-rant about the lumps in my arms, my near crippling fear of getting blown up by ISIS, the leaf blowers, and the sheer frivolousness of saying fuck-all to my life in New York and traipsing around the world.

"It's like the past six months ripped me open," I blubber, wiping away ever-present tears with the loose end of a roll of toilet paper, "like I've been hit by a car and I keep getting run over by another car, but no one can finish me off. And now I'm left to watch myself rot on the road. So what if I won a stupid cooking competition. It was a distraction at best."

Alan does not indulge my rant. "I get how *Chopped* is a stupid cooking competition. In some ways, that's true. But it's still a big deal because patterns were broken. You didn't freeze. You didn't have a breakdown on national television. You didn't come in second. You came in first. You won. Bottom line is a pattern changed."

"The producers made the decision in the end," I argue. "Besides, it didn't change the core issue. I was depressed before and I'm still depressed now. At best, the adrenaline gave me one night of bliss, but the afterglow of triumph has long since worn off. I feel like I've regressed."

"I don't think so," Alan says. "I see this happen all the time. We're going layer by layer. People seem to get a little better as we work through the superficial stuff. Not that the issues are superficial, but we have to get through the obvious first. As we go deeper, it hurts more because we're getting closer to the root issue, and people think that means they're regressing, when in reality it means we're making progress. The struggle is a map. It tells us where to look. So let's do some compassion statements and see what we find. Okay?"

"Okay," I say, hoping he's right.

Alan asks me to imagine reaching inside myself with my left hand, pulling out the depressed and terrified consciousness inside of me, and placing it across from myself. I've learned to trust him, so I close my eyes and see myself reaching in. I pull out a man who is still conscious, but necrotizing from the waist down. Alan instructs me to focus on this man, to pour compassion into every dying part of him. The familiar warmth of this process fills me as my mind begins to buzz.

"I'm so sorry nothing changes everything."

The man is scared. He is thin. He tripped and fell onto a colony of fire ants.

"I'm so sorry no matter what happens outside, you feel the same inside."

He tries to escape but he can't.

"I'm so sorry nothing you tried worked."

He is covered in insects.

"I'm so sorry you're trapped."

It was an accident.

"I'm so sorry you want to rip apart the universe but you can't."

Something awful is going to happen.

"I'm so sorry you want to burn everything down but you can't."

He is powerless to fix it.

"I'm so sorry you can't protect yourself."

There are too many of them.

"I'm so sorry they make your blood boil."
He hurts so much.
"I'm so sorry you stumbled into this mess."
They're all over him now.
"I'm so sorry it all ended this way."
There's no going back.
"I'm so sorry you lost everything."
His body is burning.
"I'm so sorry it's hard to breathe."
His body is numb.
"I'm so sorry you can't save yourself."
He couldn't say "goodbye."
"I'm so sorry it went the wrong way."
He couldn't hug them again.
"I'm so sorry there's nothing to be done about it."
It can't be undone.
"I'm so sorry you can't experience the rest of that life."
They eat him clean to the bone.

"This man," Alan whispers after a long bout of silence, "it's interesting that he comes up when he did because here is this mental image of a person who left in the middle of these loose ends, and here you are, leaving in the middle of the life you created. What do you think we should do with him? If you're the master of the universe and can do anything for him, what do you want to do for him?"

The pile of snotty tissue grows as I blow my nose and think about what this person, this thing, is doing in my head. I feel a deep need to comfort him, to send him into the arms of love as he dies alone.

"I'd find his mom," I say, surprised at my tender answer.

"What's the equivalent here?" Alan asks. "The spirit of a mother or the spirit of a family?"

"Either one." In the embers of what I saw, this suggestion feels neither hokey nor foolish.

Alan says with tenderness, "Let's invite some light to come and find this abandoned soul and take him back to a warm place, to his family."

In my mind's eye, the bleak landscape where the man was caught begins to flood with a warm, white light. Glowing orbs enter from outside my frame of mental vision, the man's eyes widening as the orbs surround him and help him off the ground.

"Can you see the light coming in?" Alan asks.

"Yes."

"Soothe him, comfort him, cry with him."

And I do.

~~~~~~~~~~~~~

I am home alone in the morning when I get an email from my dermatologist in New York with the subject line "Path Report." There is no message in the email, just an attachment from the dermatopathology lab at Columbia University that says, "Microscopic description sections show skin with a blood vessel with fibrin and surrounded by an inflammatory infiltrate of lymphocytes. Microscopic diagnosis: the changes are suggestive of nodular vasculitis." And then a note scribbled from the dermatopathologist to my dermatologist: "Please call me about this."

I Google "nodular vasculitis." The internet says it is a loosely defined term used for conditions that cause nodules on the legs, often due to inflammation of the blood vessels typically resulting from a "hypersensitivity response to tuberculosis or its antigens."

"What the fuck?" I mutter and call my dermatologist.

"I think you need to see a specialist and get some blood tests before you leave," she says. "The biopsy can only tell us so much. Look, I don't think it's serious. But there's something going on. Go see a specialist. Have them order a full blood test with a complete blood count, metabolic panel, thyroid panel, coagulation panel, and—write this down—an ANA test. See what it says, okay?"

"Okay." I gulp and drop my head into my hands. I have no idea how I'm going to find a doctor who will see me on such short notice. My American health insurance has been cancelled and my international insurance doesn't kick in until four days after I arrive in Malaysia.

If I even get to Malaysia. Maybe this whole Remote Year thing was just a string on the universal puppet show, designed to get me out of New York and back to Reno just in time to get sick. Really sick. Not depressed sick, but physically sick.

My mother calls in a favor fifteen years in the making, from one of my father's best friends.

"Dr. Jack Morgan," she says to me. "He led the pack of motorcycles at your father's funeral. Your father meant a lot to him. He's going to see you even though you're uninsured. Eight a.m. tomorrow."

When I arrive at Dr. Morgan's office, the receptionist hands me a chart to fill out. I am halfway through the chart when the nurse calls for me and takes me to the back.

"I haven't finished filling this out," I say.

"Don't worry about it," Dr. Morgan says, swooping in. "I know who you are."

He takes me into an exam room, listens to my chest, finds the beat of my heart, studies the lumps. He is quiet, clinical, but when he brings his hand to my chin and takes a good look at my face, I swear I see the faint glassiness of tears in his eyes.

"What are you looking for?" I ask.

"Redness," he says, and looks away.

Dr. Morgan calls in a nurse to take my blood, and tells me the results will be back in a few days. When I try to pay him, he refuses and tells me it's taken care of. "Sometimes I still miss him," he says.

"Me too."

He calls two days later.

"The lab results are a little inconclusive," he tells me. "The good news is it's not anything serious. Your white blood cell counts are fine; there's no indication of cancer or anything like that."

A disconcerting combination of release and irritation washes over me. I'm relieved to know it's not something serious, but annoyed that the results are otherwise vague.

Dr. Morgan continues, "Your ANA levels are a bit elevated, and typically when we see that combined with the skin irritations, we think lupus. But your ANA isn't off the chart. And there isn't a conclusive test or treatment for lupus anyway. Honestly, I think this was triggered by stress. The best thing you can do is get those stress levels down."

Because it's that easy.

"I'm supposed to get on a one-way flight to Malaysia in two weeks."

Tell me not to get on the plane. Tell me you don't recommend it, that now is not a good time.

"Sounds like an adventure."

"Or an extremely stupid decision."

Make the choice for me. Tell me what to do.

"I don't see why you can't leave," Dr. Morgan says. "If symptoms get worse, just come home."

I sigh.

"One more thing, Dr. Morgan. Can you tell me what my thyroid levels look like?"

I hear him adjust the phone against his ear and shuffle through the lab reports.

"Your thyroid levels look good. Totally normal."

"Huh," I mumble. "Well, thank you. Again. I appreciate all this."

"You're welcome. I'm glad I'm still around to do it."

I hang up the phone, rest my chin in my hand. *My thyroid is functioning without the levothyroxine.*

I always knew my physical body could function without the antidepressants. My mind might crumble, but my somatic system would still operate. I assumed the hypothyroidism needed synthetic hormones to stay in balance and would be a lifelong ailment always requiring medication. My grandfather had a low-functioning thyroid, so no one was surprised when the hypothyroid diagnosis popped up along with everything else. When I dumped my levothyroxine in a frenzy back in New York, I figured the clumps of hair falling out, the excruciating charley horses, the always cold-to-the-bone would return and send me right back to the pharmacy where I'd refill my two generic, seven-dollar prescriptions and never abandon the levothyroxine again. But symptoms didn't return. And now I know why: My thyroid has righted itself.

Maybe, just maybe, my mind will too.

13

I blink and I am back at the Reno airport. Under the desert sun, my mother watches as I unload my suitcase and two backpacks from the trunk. I take them out at a glacial pace, trying to slow down time.

"I'm in no state to be doing this," I tell her.

"It's not too late to back out. You don't have to get on the plane if you don't want to," my mother says.

Despite it all, my throat tightens at the idea of staying in Reno. Getting on the plane might mean pouring gas on my psyche and lighting a match, but the shame of not getting on the plane is stronger than the shame of cracking in a foreign country.

"Will you be able to call me when you get there?" my mother asks.

"At the very least I can send an email when I get to Wi-Fi," I tell her.

I check the car once. Twice. There is nothing left to do but leave.

My mother takes my face in her hands. "You're better now than when you arrived. I can see it in your eyes."

I don't know if I believe her, but I try to pretend. I fight to hold back tears and keep my composure, latching on tight to one last embrace.

In San Francisco, I see a currency-exchange booth in the airport and dig through my wallet to convert whatever dollars I have left. I hand the cashier a single ten-dollar bill and she gives me a stack of brightly colored notes and a handful of coins that fatten my small wallet, a total of forty Malaysian ringgits. I tuck the wallet into a backpack hanging over my front. With one pack on my back and another slung over my belly, I look like a pregnant turtle. I am stuffed with cameras and hard drives and toiletries. Vaccination reports and official documents and backup credit cards. A mug. A journal. A clothesline. A change of clothes and a pile of snacks and two Ambien in a plastic bag.

"For the plane, to sleep," an old friend told me as he handed me the parting gift. Other than a packet of malaria pills and a small supply of anti-diarrhea capsules, they are the only drug I bring with me. And yet I know I will not take the Ambien. I keep it as a talisman, a reminder of what I left behind.

I wander through the San Francisco terminal, tired and puffy-eyed. I remember that 5,538 days ago, my mother and I were in this same airport, waiting on standby for a flight to take us home to my father. I look around for the spot where I rested my head on her shoulder and she told me it was "just you and me, baby." But nothing jogs my memory. The airport, my body, my mind—it has all been bulldozed and redesigned.

~~~~~~~~

I am over open sea. A flight attendant scolds me for using my phone and insists I turn it off and put it away. No phones allowed on Chinese airlines, she tells me, not even in airplane mode. Then she reaches across me and slams my window shade shut. I look around and see my male, Chinese cabinmates swiping away with their shades up while flight attendants walk past. Three hours before we land, the same attendant takes away my airline headphones, turns off my in-flight entertainment, and puts my window shade up without explanation. The Chinese men keep watching their movies and chuckling over their drinks.

Be less space.

I pull a blanket over my legs and sink into my seat, curling up into a ball and resting my forehead against the window. Eight hours out of the United States and I'm already getting in trouble, already getting lost in translation.

Left with nothing but myself, I watch Earth change below me. Smog hangs above the ocean like a suffocating blanket. When the haze breaks, blue ocean does not appear. Instead the ocean is a sea of brick, miles and miles of red brushed with light strokes of wavy white. Suddenly land appears, with lush greens and tropical woods reaching toward the horizon. Golf courses and windmills and estates pepper the hazy, green earth. Nuclear power plants bellow pure, white steam into the atmosphere. Acres-wide buildings stretch from one end of my field of vision to the other. Animal processing plants and sweatshops. One after the other. Yet from 35,000 feet above, the world below seems so peaceful. Just like I know that from the outside, this trip looks like nothing but gilded opportunity.

Alan once asked me, "What would it mean to get through this year? What would that look like?"

I didn't know how to answer then, when the trip seemed so far away. I spent every day just scraping through to get here, to get to this moment on the plane. Now I am here, suspended halfway between what was and what will be.

I keep my expectations low. I expect to be uncomfortable. I expect to not like everyone in the group. I expect to eat some damn delicious food. But my expectations end there. I can't ask for what I want—clarity, healing, joy, a relationship, money, a new career—no, I can't burden myself with the expectation of all of that. The letdown would be too great. All I know is if I make it through this year, my life will never be the same. That is the only reason why I'm on this plane. Because after this, it will be different. It must be different.

After a long layover in Shanghai and another six-hour flight, it is one in the morning when I step out of Malaysian customs into the dead of the Kuala Lumpur International Airport. Not a soul stands behind the counter, and my fellow passengers walk on by without a shrug. I tuck my head and follow the last person through until we are spit out into an empty mall that scatters travelers in every direction. All the storefronts are closed, but neon signs light up for Auntie Anne's Pretzels, Sunglass Hut, and The Coffee Bean & Tea Leaf. For a moment it feels like I'm still in New York, somewhere in the doldrums of the Manhattan Mall on 34th Street, like I've traveled all around the world just to go nowhere at all.

I pick a direction and walk until I find a sign with a bright-white, bed-shaped icon and an arrow pointing to KLIA2, the airport's second terminal. I have a cot in KLIA2's capsule hotel to get me through the night, since I don't meet up with Remote Year until tomorrow. After two full days of planes and airports, I need a shower and a mattress before I introduce myself to seventy-three new travel companions.

I follow the signs across to the other side of the airport where the AirTran to KLIA2 picks up, only to discover that it doesn't run this late at night. I look around for an airport employee, but still, I am alone.

I double back and follow the little taxi transportation icons across the airport, back through the mall, down a few escalators, and into a group of men smoking near an exit. I roll my suitcase up to them and say, "KLIA2?" They take drags from their cigarettes and stare back at me, without answering. I hold up my phone and point to the name of the airport hotel. One of them gestures toward a taxi stand around the corner.

"KLIA2?" I ask the man behind the counter, attempting to confirm that the taxi driver will take me to the right place.

The man nods and charges me two Malaysian ringgits, about fifty cents. "You pay driver the rest," he grunts, and points me back toward the group of men.

I return to the drivers, this time waving my receipt. One of them steps out from the crowd and signals me to follow him outside. We step into a haze of humidity and smog that sucks my clothes to my body like a plastic-wrapped supermarket chicken. When I try to take my first breath, I choke on a lungful of smoke.

"Indonesia," the driver says, loading my bags into the back of a beat-up red sedan. "They burn many tree. Many forest."

He opens the back door for me and I clear my throat and climb in. The air is so thick the lampposts glow like fuzzy orbs suspended over the street, passing by us slowly until we pick up speed. So much speed. We are not at the airport anymore. Suddenly we are on the highway, rushing away from the terminal into the misty darkness. I sit up straighter in my seat and look out the window for signs of civilization. But the night is saturated with smoke and humidity.

Did the man not understand when I said KLIA2? I try to think back but my head is as thick as the air outside. I haven't slept in two days and it's like my interaction with the taxi driver from five minutes ago has fallen out of my head, so I just sit there and watch the meter tick through five, ten, fifteen ringgits.

I am in a strange car with a strange man at two in the morning in a strange country.

Eighteen, nineteen, twenty.

I do not have cell-phone service and no one knows where I am and I never learned how to throw a punch and twenty-one, twenty-two. Ten more minutes pass and my heart beats faster and outside the windows is nothing but dark and *I am alone in this car* and twenty-three, twenty-four.

Tourists get abducted.

Twenty-five.

Women are sold into sex slavery.

Twenty-six.

I am powerless.

Twenty-seven.

I close my eyes and see myself opening the door and rolling out of the car while it is moving. I see myself scraped up, walking on the highway. I see the taxi driver pulling into a Kuala Lumpur slum and forcing me out of the car, into his lair. I see him pulling into downtown Kuala Lumpur and dropping me off, nothing more than a little miscommunication between us. I see myself without enough money to pay him, and he takes my bag, passport, and phone. He strips me of my lifelines and leaves me, alone.

Twenty-eight.

My mother's voice: *"For God's sake, if I had an intuition that something was going to happen, I wouldn't let you go."*

Twenty-nine.

"You've handled everything that's come at you so far. I always trust you to handle it."

Thirty.

I choose to believe her.

Thirty-one, thirty-two.

Whatever happens, whatever is happening, I will handle it.

Thirty-three, thirty-four.

I lock eyes with the driver in the rearview mirror and look for any sign of danger in the face staring back at me.

"KLIA2?" I ask without breaking my gaze.

"Yes, yes! Very far!"

And with that the lights of KLIA2 appear.

Thirty-five.

I exhale and melt into the seat. The meter ticks to thirty-six ringgits as we pull into the terminal. I have thirty-seven ringgits and change.

I give the man everything I have.

~~~~~~~~~~~~~~~~~

My heart rate slows only when the water hits me. The patter of the lukewarm droplets drowns out the snores of other weary travelers, their guttural rumbles hidden behind thin curtains that pull across each four-by-eight-foot bunk in the capsule hotel. I am wide awake, adrenaline still pulsing through me from the innocuous taxi ride that, for a moment, went so wrong in my head.

In fact it all went right, down to the exact amount of cash I needed to pay the driver. The whole trip went right. No missed connections. No issues going through customs. No screaming babies seated next to me. Even the airplane food wasn't all bad. When the flight attendant took my drink and turned off my TV and made me put my phone away, I didn't fight. There wasn't any point. Because I didn't fight, I didn't get angry. I simply let it be.

I handled it. And I handled the taxi ride, too.

The shower water turns cool, but I don't get out. I want to feel this clarity, of handling the situation and coming out just fine. It seems so basic, so obvious—and yet this new awareness has shattered a pattern that has gripped me since I got off the Effexor 182 days ago. For a moment, I am proud of myself.

Still, I'm not sure where antidepressant withdrawal ends and I begin. Maybe there is no obvious line to cross. All I know is I was dead for so long and now I am stuffed with worry and regret. But even bubbling with fear, today I chose to let it be. Whatever comes next. Whatever appears. Today I let it be.

14

Remote Year Libertatum is a motley crew. We are not only from a colorful United States, but Australia, Belgium, Canada, Greece, New Zealand, Russia, Poland, Serbia, the United Kingdom, and the Virgin Islands. One of us has never left the state of Virginia. Another hasn't had a permanent address in seven years. Our youngest is twenty-four, the oldest in her early fifties. The tallest is six-foot-six and the shortest scrapes five feet. Some aren't sure if their jobs will survive a year of remote work. At least two people straight up lie to their companies and don't disclose that they are working on the other side of the world. The ones who don't doubt their job security are software developers or self-employed. The rest are mostly marketers, recruiters, and graphic designers. We have one matchmaker, one architect, and one guy who owns the most expensive gas station in the United States. It's the last gas station between the Orlando airport and Disney World. Prices are triple the national average. The owner says he lost 80 percent of his customers when he jacked up prices, but it doesn't matter, because European tourists rushing from Disney World to fill up their rental cars before they get to the airport don't know the difference. Three days after we arrive, the gas station owner decides the Remote Year apartment complex where we are all housed is too dingy, the towels too scratchy, and the service not up to par. He books out the rest of the month at one of Kuala Lumpur's luxury hotels and invites select members of the group to swim in the rooftop infinity pool.

We have one devout Jehovah's Witness, three Bible thumpers, one outspoken atheist, two cancer survivors, and one ex-wife of a no-name NBA player. She comes down with a mystery parasite within the first few days of arriving, goes to the hospital, and never returns to the group. We have one vegan who doesn't drink and more than a few functioning alcoholics. One of them funnels his arrival anxiety into a bottle of vodka and tries to make mac and cheese without removing the stove's protective glass cover. He creates an explosion of molten glass and hot cheese at 4:00 a.m. and shows up to our group orientation all banged up. When it's his turn to stand up and introduce himself, I immediately forget his name because I am too busy staring at the black eye standing out on his bald head.

With seventy-three new people to meet and seventy-three personalities to manage, the extroverts keep the group busy while the introverts, including me, plaster themselves against walls and barstools in an attempt to remain upright amid the mayhem. Every conversation is loaded with curiosity: What do you do? Why are you here? What are you passionate about? Are you going to the Maldives this weekend? Does anyone have an extra power converter I could borrow? Do we need a visa to go to Thailand? But really, what are you passionate about?

"You okay?" I hear a soft voice from behind me during one of the many get-to-know-each-other happy hours organized by Remote Year. I turn to the voice and find a tall, thin Remote with jet-black hair and square glasses. I recognize him from the Facebook group we all joined before arriving in Malaysia but can't remember his name. I only remember he had an answer for all things travel and tech and managed to turn himself into the go-to Remote Year problem-solver before we even showed up. Phone not working from country to country? Go to Settings > Cellular > (Roaming On) > Cellular Data Network > Cellular Data APN = h2g2. Not sure about the Cambodian visa requirements? Don't bother with the online system. Just get it on arrival for thirty dollars, but don't forget to bring dollars (they only take USD) and extra passport photos. Trying to figure out which credit card to apply for to maximize points? Go for the Citi Preferred and Chase Sapphire lines, with a Charles Schwab debit. No foreign transaction fees and they don't gouge you on the points exchange.

"I'm Ross," the man says, and holds out one hand while taking a sip of his drink with the other.

The nodules in my arms throb as we shake.

"You okay?" he asks again. "You look a little overwhelmed."

"That about sums it up," I say. "It's just a lot. I do better with smaller groups. Or no groups."

"I have a solution."

"What's that?"

"Alcohol." Ross smirks, takes a sip of his drink, and winces. "Malaysian wine is terrible."

I smile and peek into his cup.

"May I?" I ask.

Ross hands me the plastic cup. I swirl it, stick my nose in for a whiff, then take a sip. The wine tastes like sour grape juice cut with ethanol.

"Oh good god, that's awful." I give Ross back his cup and grab an untouched cracker from someone's abandoned plate to kill the lingering taste on my tongue.

"You look like you know what you're talking about when it comes to wine," Ross says.

"I do. Sort of. I'm a professional chef."

"Oh you're the chef! Someone mentioned there was a chef in the group."

"That's me. What do you do?"

"Software developer. And then I work at the suicide hotline at night."

"That's . . . huh . . . that's good of you." I stumble over my words and don't know what to say. I never once even thought about calling the suicide hotline. It simply never crossed my mind as I was calculating the velocity of a falling object from thirty floors above.

"It felt like the right thing to do," Ross says. "Anyway, if you ever want to cook, I brought a chef's knife with me."

"Smart. I didn't even think to do that."

Ross shrugs. "I figured I wouldn't want to go out to eat all the time," he says.

We both stare at the horde of strangers chatting in front of us.

"Okay, I'm going to go back in there and mingle," he says.

"Good luck," I say.

Ross downs the rest of his wine and takes a deep breath. "See you around," he says, and disappears into the crowd.

~~~~~~~~~~

I try to slip away from the group, to find pockets of solitude, but there is no peace to be found in Kuala Lumpur. At all waking hours and around every corner, a new building is being constructed, an old street getting torn up. When jet lag gets me up at 5:00 a.m., I take a walk and try to find some quiet. But street vendors are already up and tinkering and when they sweep the sidewalk they do it with a broom made of sticks and the sound grates and I cover my ears with my hands and run back to my assigned apartment.

Nobody else is bothered. There are seventy-three other Remotes and none of them seem to notice. They tune it out and go about their day, stuffing their faces with street-side dumplings and roti while a sidewalk is bulldozed beside them. But I feel every hit. It is as if the construction shows up just for me, to remind me that despite the work I've done, despite the days I've counted, despite the raindrops I've felt, I, too, am still just a pile of smoldering wreckage. Day after day there is no relief from the noise, the input. I don't get used to it. I don't adjust. It's like I am infected by this place, the constant swirls of sound and smog and smells seeping into my body, assaulting my senses, destroying my patience.

Is this still lingering withdrawal?

I sit at a table in the corner of the Remote Year provided workspace, staring out the window at a half-built tangle of metal across the street. The window is razor-thin and I can hear every hammer, every screech, so I shove silicone plugs into my ears and put on noise-cancelling headphones. I can still hear bang, bang, bang so I stream static brown noise through the headphones. Brown noise, specifically, seems to cancel out the higher frequencies that light my nerves on fire. The whole setup finally drowns out the banging and I find a moment of peace. Artificial peace.

Across the room, a local named Nik begins to unpack plastic take-out containers of food. A round man with a rounder face that seems to always hold a smile and a giggle, Nik was born in Malaysia and works as part of the Remote Year Kuala Lumpur city team. It is his job to deal with any issues that come up, from fixing faulty Wi-Fi routers to planning group events to giving directions to the city's best late-night curry. He is on-call twenty-four hours a day and yet never seems flustered, never complains. Not even when he's sweeping shards of glass off a drunken Remote's floor in the wee hours of the morning.

I pause the brown noise, take off my headphones, take out my earplugs, and wander over to where Nik is arranging a box of crispy, fried-sesame balls on a plate.

"These are local Malaysian breakfast street food called *kuih bom*," he tells me. "They're made of a sort of sticky rice with mung beans in the inside. They are gone by seven, eight in the morning. You want to try, lah?"

Nik speaks a creole called Manglish, a delightful mashup of Malay and English that eliminates nonessential words and punctuates phrases with a perky "lah."

I nod, welcoming the culinary distraction. Nik hands me one of the golf-ball sized pastries. The golden exterior crunches gently against the chewy, glutinous rice dough stuffed with a sweet and earthy paste.

"These are mung beans?" I ask. "They're so sweet."

"Actually, this is considered a savory breakfast. We Kelantanese and Terengganuians of Northeast Malaysia are known for our sweet tooth. We put condensed milk on everything, lah." Nik breaks into a wide smile and rubs his bulbous belly.

I finish the *kuih bom* and wipe the residual fry grease off my hands, wondering if there are any fresh vegetables around that aren't deep-fried or covered in sugar.

"How are you settling into Kuala Lumpur so far?" Nik asks. A handsaw whirs somewhere in the building and I consider my answer, not wanting to offend the man who calls this place home.

"It's loud here," I say, forgetting the vegetables and taking another *kuih bom*. "I'm having trouble dealing with the noise."

"I know. They are building, building, building. This is sort of a new thing, over the past ten years. Suddenly, boom! Skyscrapers everywhere. We just get used to it."

"Teach me your powers because I can't seem to get used to it. Is there anywhere quiet around here?"

Nik laughs. "Aiya! Maybe not in KL proper. But if you go outside the city it is quiet. Jungles and lots of green, up in the mountains. If you go to the north, there is a town called Sekinchan near the sea. It is kilometers and kilometers of rice paddies. Nothing to do up there. But you can have a kilo of shrimp for a few ringgits and stare at rice paddies in silence."

There is a crash across the street at the construction site, followed by a symphony of electric saws. My eyes fill with tears and I can't be in the room any longer.

"I'm sorry. I have to go. Thank you for the sesame balls. I just . . . I just can't listen to this anymore."

I pack up my things and say goodbye and rush back to my apartment. I head straight for the bathroom and begin to fill the bath with water the color of lukewarm tea. Old pipes, I hope. I let the water run, the bathroom walls and the pounding water muffling the sounds of construction outside. The water turns clear and I strip down and get in. I can still feel the noise pounding into my body. I dunk my head under the water and everything goes quiet. I come up for air and it's roaring again. I fill the bathtub to the brim, sink back down, rest my head on the lip of the bathtub. My ears fall below the water line, eyes, nose, and mouth barely peeking through the surface. If I am still, I can breathe and it is quiet. I close my eyes. Don't move. Sleep.

~~~~~~~~~~~~~~~

On the morning of Sunday, September 11, I wake up to a message from Nik. He wants to know if I want to run an errand with him and a friend in the Malaysian highlands. It is their day off, and they need to drop off a kitchen trolley cart for a wedding. "Then we will wait around for the wedding to finish and pick the trolley up again. Maybe grab lunch. It will be quiet and calm. This isn't a Remote Year official outing, but I thought you might need to get away, lah."

I don't understand wasting a precious day off just to deliver and wait around for a single kitchen trolley, but then again I don't understand most of this country. Nothing works with any sort of efficiency or logic. Air conditioners break, but maintenance doesn't bother to show up. Automatic hand dryers are plugged in and turned on, but bathroom attendants inexplicably don't let you use them. Individual paper napkins are wrapped in individual envelopes of plastic and you get a receipt for everything. A receipt for buying a banana. A receipt for using the restroom. Three receipts for a single credit-card purchase. When four people order breakfast and coffee, the waiter brings two people their coffee before their food, but the other two people don't get their coffee until after the food arrives. And when the other two coffees finally do show up, it's tea. And then some guy with a cement cutter shows up and starts hacking at the sidewalk and the sound pulls the color out of my face and my stomach turns to knots and I get dizzy and sprint away from the restaurant, leaving everyone at the table confused.

Nik is right. I need to get out of here.

I meet Nik and his friend, Yong, at a café and watch them scarf down white toast spread thick with sticky coconut jam and served alongside half-boiled eggs soaked in soy sauce. I sip a frosty iced *cham*, a Malaysian concoction of coffee and tea swirled together with sweetened condensed milk. The café's stale air hangs with fry oil and sweat, and my skin prickles with heat. The clinks of spoons on porcelain and the clang of pots on stoves ring in my ears like an orchestra of gunshots. Though the café is dim, the lights are bright and I am somehow both blinded and struggling to see at the same time. I get a little dizzy, but I can't run away from here. I don't want to embarrass myself in front of these two kind strangers carting me along on their day off, so I force myself to focus on the bright-yellow egg yolks mingling with pools of soy. The *cham* sits on my tongue, thick and dull.

Yong is just as tall and wide as Nik and with the three of us stuffed into the car, its small frame sinks under our weight. They roll down the windows and each light a cigarette, sending both smoke and smog rushing in one window and out the other as we speed down the highway and out of the Kuala Lumpur city limits. We pull farther and farther away from the city and into clear skies and my spirits begin to lift, as if all the polluted energy inside me stuck to the haze and lingered on the horizon behind us. As we gain elevation and the landscape changes from gray concrete and ruddy sprawl to lush green canopies and forest, I stick my torso out the back window and let the cool, clear air calm my body. After an hour we arrive at the wedding venue and drop off the kitchen trolley. We are told to come back in four or five hours, so we get back in the car and drive.

We park the car on the side of a dirt road and hike through a small village to a river running brown with silt. Abandoned huts and shaded, wooden decks line the water. Rain begins to fall just as we arrive, sending the three of us to huddle under a covered deck and wait for the rain to pass or the caterer to call, whichever comes first. I lie down on the warped wood and swat at mosquitos, my layer of DEET from the morning already sweating off.

"Mosquis like the taste of white blood," Nik giggles as he takes a drag off his cigarette.

"A foreign delicacy," Yong says, thumping down on the deck. "Speaking of which. What should we eat for lunch?"

"You just had breakfast," I say.

"We Malays are always thinking about what we eat next. You must do as we do, Brooke," Yong says before resting his hands over his protruding belly and nodding off to sleep.

"There are three main ethnic groups in Malaysia," Nik adds. "Malay, Chinese, and Indian. Our food, like our culture, is a fusion of all those groups. Like the mosquis want to eat you, we have to eat it all!"

"I feel like I've been nauseous since I got here," I say, curling into a ball. "It's like I've been infected. Like I'm possessed by some sort of . . . ickiness."

"Maybe you are. Kuala Lumpur is full of spirits, you know. Many of them are bad spirits, evil spirits." Nik puts out his cigarette and settles himself on the deck.

"Say more about that."

"Back in the day, before Islam came in the fourteenth century, we used to be a Hindu state. The Hindu religion, you know, believes in a lot of entities and multi-gods. It became part of our culture, in a sense. The spirits in the stones, the spirits in the trees. And if you think about it, this part of Asia is very primordial, so we have spirits going back thousands of years. Angry spirits that are not like your modern, I'm-a-turn-of-the-century-gentleman-now-I'm-going-to-haunt-your-hotel spirit. No, this is some crazy shit!" Nik looks at me without a hint of jest.

"I was in an Uber the other day," I say, "and the driver refused to take a particular exit because he said it was full of ghosts. And the concierge at our apartment complex told me the building is haunted."

"It's real, yo! I've felt it." Nik's eyebrows raise so high, they seem to merge with his hairline.

"Have you ever been to New York, Nik?" I ask.

"I have not. I would like to."

"Today is the anniversary of 9/11."

"It is." Nik nods.

"If you ever make it there you should go to Ground Zero. Then you should call me afterward and tell me what you think of it. The memorial is built on top of where the Twin Towers stood, so there are two black squares spanning the foundations, with water falling into the center. I avoid going down to that area. The closer I get to it, the more trapped I feel. Like I'm being squeezed tighter and tighter as I approach it. I wasn't even in New York in 2001. I didn't know anyone who died that day. But it's like the sorrow, the oppression, lives there. It burrows into your soul."

"And what do you feel here in Kuala Lumpur?" Nik asks.

I look around. There are green trees and a brown river. A hazy sky swollen with thunderclouds. Brilliant orange birds of paradise sway in the wind and a stray black-and-white cat hops from rock to rock. Empty plastic bottles line the riverbank and deflated balloons hang limp from a bridge. I look back to Nik, who is smoking again.

"Like the light is no match for the darkness."

Nik nods with understanding. "We have local shamans in our culture. If anyone ever builds over an area, whether it's Chinese, Malay, or Indian, there's a cleansing ceremony led by the shamans. It's tied to our local Malay martial arts, known as Silat. It's something like jujitsu, but with a spiritual side to it. You're not just defending yourself physically, you're also defending yourself spiritually. So you may have two shamans, one who is Chinese and one who is Indian, but they're both versed in the Silat. And it's all mixed with Islamic customs. They work together to cleanse whatever spirits hang around." He takes a drag and exhales. "Maybe we need to teach you some Silat."

"I could use some Silat."

"Think about it," Nik continues. "KL is less than 200 years old, lah, which is not as old as most American cities. To think it started in the jungle, at the confluence of two rivers as wooden huts, and it grew and grew and grew and now it's sprawl with concrete buildings and alleyways and side streets. As the city grew, we had to cut down forest. When the shamans of old days cleansed the area, they bottled up the spirits and then threw the bottle into the woods. But as the city sprawled, what used to be a spiritual dumping ground now has an apartment on it." Nik goes quiet for a few moments. The trickle of the river and the patter of rain on the covered deck fill the silence. "I hate thinking about the supernatural. It makes me feel out of control."

Nik settles himself down for a nap while I turn my attention to the idea of constructing life on the foundation of death. This is the only thing we humans have mastered, I reckon. We like to run around thinking we are the rulers of our fate, that we choose what to believe in and how to live our lives. What agency do we have, really, when our entire system is built on those who came before us and those who came before them and those who came before them?

Two months and eight days after my father died, the Twin Towers fell and the massacre was declared a terrorist act. My mother turned to me and said, "Your father wouldn't have liked this. He was still in the Reserves during the Gulf War, after the first World Trade Center bombing. When that happened, he told me if he was called to serve, he was going to go. And that there would be no discussion. For all his faults, he was a protector."

My mother and I stood together, watching the Twin Towers fall, silently asking ourselves a series of questions that would take years to answer. *Did anyone know this was going to happen? Were there warning signs we missed? What's happening to our world? Now what?* My father was gone, left to mingle with whatever was left of the 2,977 souls that died on that September Tuesday. He couldn't protect us anymore, but he couldn't shatter us either. Our world came to a stop along with everyone else's and hovered as a new history began, just waiting for us to exhale before reversing direction and picking up speed.

I adjust myself on the patio, splinters of dried wood digging into my skin. Nik and Yong snore gently, so easily lulled to sleep with nothing to do. I can't sleep. So I trace back through the decisions that led me here, trying to find the pivotal moment that brought me to this rickety deck on the banks of a brown Malaysian river. I go back, starting with eating the *kuih bom*, back through Dr. Morgan telling me I was healthy enough to get on the plane. I go back to New York, to the moment I put the Remote Year deposit down on my credit card. I go to the window. And to what led me there. I go back to the bakery, to the late-night fights and the burns that stung and the cuts that bled. I go back to the burning stomach and leg cramps that plagued me before my bile reflux and hypothyroidism diagnosis. Back to watching the Twin Towers fall. Back to the taxi driver who sped through Naples at midnight to get my mother and me to the airport so we could catch the last flight out of Italy and get to my father. I go back to when I thought he was immortal.

I lose the single thread in a tangled messy mass of life before death. I can't see an end to it, can't figure out who is responsible for it. So what brought me here? Was it the antidepressant withdrawal, or was it me? Who bent that ironing board in half? Did I do it? Or did my father loosen the hinges decades before, when he walked out of the door with a loaded shotgun, blind with rage? Or did it begin when my grandfather threw my father into a burning fireplace? And what of his father? And his? What of the pain that seems to come from nowhere, sticking inside me and pulling me down to a non-functioning cave of anxiety and desperation begging for relief in any form—food, booze, medication—could this simply be generations of sorrow, centuries of grief, that have reached a tipping point I can no longer ignore? Just like we can only stand so much heat before we begin to sweat, can we only stand so much grief before it must find a way out? Because all of this feels a lot like mourning. Raw, confusing, unpredictable, rage-filled mourning. Who wants to feel that when you can feel your throat close around a little, blue pill instead?

One pill—or even 32,760—is no match for the entire history of our humanity. And yet the only other choice is to face it all, feel it all. I'm not sure I'm strong enough. Already this process has broken me down, my soul falling through a skinned and bloody carcass left for vultures. But there is still something simmering inside me; I can feel it. It is dark enough that, despite the work I've done, it still poisons me from the inside out.

A clap of thunder booms overhead, startling Nik and Yong from their nap. Nik looks at his watch. The trolley will not be ready for pickup for a few more hours, but the covered deck won't protect us from the sudden onslaught of sideways rain.

Raindrops dripping off his beard, Nik breaks into a wide smile and says, "Lunch?"

Yong pats his belly and nods. "I must pray first," he says, referring to the five daily prayers of his Muslim heritage.

"Let us go to the car for some shelter and then we will pray and eat," Nik says, looking at me. "Sound good, lah?"

I nod and gather my things, not bothering to shelter myself from the rain. I am already wet, and we have a long walk back to the car. The only way out is through.

15

I wake up in my Kuala Lumpur apartment, the morning light fighting a losing battle with the darkness of the expansive room. The once cream-colored carpet is spotted with mysterious splatter and the walls are browned with streaks converging on a plaid headboard the color of vomit. The air conditioning whirs and blows anemic-but-cool air into the space. Patches of dark mold crawl around the unit. But it is so stifling hot and humid here in Malaysia that I am okay with risking exposure to whatever is growing on the walls in exchange for the relief of the air conditioning.

I roll over and imagine the weight of my energy mingling with the heavy, humid particles in the room. Maybe the air conditioning will filter my energy too. Maybe it will engulf it, recycle it, and spit it out fresh and clean and cool. Maybe the walls will absorb it and trap it here along with the others who inhabited this space before me. Though I am alone and this bedroom is twice the size of my New York City apartment, this room somehow feels crowded with all the souls who came before, like this apartment, this city, is where souls get caught on their way from whatever life is to whatever death becomes. The ashen figures of Pompeii. The incinerated heartbeats of 9/11. My father. Anyone whose life was interrupted by dark serendipity. They are all here, trapped in the pulse of the living.

They appear to me as a sort of deep knowing. The sort of knowing that lingers behind after someone leaves a room and you can still feel their presence in the air. They are the feeling of standing in the presence of evil, of walking into an unfamiliar room and sensing something terrible once happened within its walls. They are unbound, neglected freedom looking for guidance in a body. And I am a perfectly shattered host.

They seem to whisper from deep within me.

"We are lonely among so many."

I get up and splash water on my face.

"We are lonely. Set us free."

They watch me move through the thick Malaysian air and whisper:

"We are the strata hanging low above the horizon."

I get out of bed and look at myself in the mirror. The circles under my eyes are dark and my skin is tanned but sallow. It is not jet lag. It is not something I ate. Is all of this the depression creeping back up, like Dr. Chin said it might? I rack my brain for the number of days since I last took a Wellbutrin, but my head is muddled and can't find the number. I count the months on my fingers. April. May. June. July. August. Five months. Maybe.

The alarm on my phone goes off. It is 7:55 a.m. At eight the noise begins. *Get out.*

I pick up speed and dot concealer under my eyes and brush my cheeks with blush. I throw my hair into a bun and wash my armpits with soap—*there is no time for a shower*—and cover myself in a layer of sunscreen and a cloud of DEET. I go to make my bed—*don't bother with the bed*—find shorts, a shirt, my shoes. *Where is my other shoe?* I turn around looking for the shoe and it is under my bed and when I kneel down to grab it, the noise begins.

Outside my window, two men with jackhammers and concrete saws don't so much construct but demolish a large pile of cement. They string a few extension cords from a crumbling building and cut through chunks of concrete for seemingly no reason at all. When I arrived, I asked the doorman what they were doing and he told me he didn't know, but that it's been going on for years and it's still a pile of rubble. At nightfall when the cacophony stops, the two men change into one of half a dozen shirts slung across plastic hangers hooked to hardened pipes. They light cigarettes, sip on cans of soda, and sleep on an old mattress behind a half-built wall. Eight a.m. comes again. They wake. They dress. They destroy.

The unnatural friction between metal and cement burrows into my chest. I grab my shoe and put in my earplugs, but they are no match for the all-encompassing pitch of machinery bellowing through my room. Instead of a jackhammer into the sidewalk it's a jackhammer into my sternum. My stomach turns to acid, and I finish dressing as fast as I can and gather my things and stuff them into my bag, but the noise is crushing me faster than I can pack. I need to get out of here, but I know it doesn't matter where I go. There are drills in cafés. Pickaxes on the streets. Handsaws in the workspace. Everywhere I go in this city there is noise and clamor and even when it stops there is traffic and there are horns and people of all nationalities recklessly crossing the streets. There are billboards and bulging trashcans and beggars. Hawkers and street vendors and lights. Ladyboys and businessmen and potholes. Poverty and wealth and malaise. New York City and Kuala Lumpur. Same same, but different.

I am infected to my core.

This was supposed to be the answer. The antidote. Get out of New York City and get out of that old life. Leave it all. Change it all. Goddamn eat, pray, love it all.

Nausea and unease ripple through my skeleton and send shards of hardened tissue into my nerves. My heart is racing and before long I can feel the nodules in my arms pulse. My blood is boiling and my arms are hot and thick and I want to carve out each node with a knife just to release the pressure trapped inside.

Get out.

I drop to a knee to put on my shoe, but it is too late. Something is happening. My arms are heavy, and looping each end of my shoelaces together takes unflinching concentration. This is not like when the New York streets turned red with blood. Or when I screamed into the night. Or when I sent pieces of the ironing board flying across the room. This is different. I can see, but my peripheral vision is fuzzy. I can hear, but even the sound of jackhammering seems far away. I can speak, but the words come a beat too late. I know where I am, but it's like I've been drugged by this space. By this room. By *them.*

I take a shallow breath and focus on tying my shoes. *Over, under, around, and through.* The laces fumble in my stiffening fingers. I might throw up. The volume turns back up and I drop my head and cover my ears with my hands. I abandon my shoe and fall to the floor. My system is in overdrive and also trying to shut down. The pressure in my arms intensifies and spreads through the rest of my body, weighing it down like molten lead.

Time slows as my head comes to a rest on the stained carpet. But this isn't about rest. I need the pressure of the floor on my temple to remind me that I am still here, that the floor is beneath me and below that the foundation of the building and below that Earth. My hands clench and release against the carpet. The rough fibers burrow into my cheek and I try to feel the force of the floor pushing back against me, but I am trapped like a cricket in a web, swaddled in a cocoon of dark energy feeding on itself until my muscles are searing and I wail an inhuman wail that doesn't belong on Earth. It is only in its lingering moments that I realize the howl was so high-pitched it barely made a sound.

The pounding outside continues, but I've lost the edges of my body, and the noise and my skin and the floor have blended into one. Unlike New York, where the force of life seemed trapped inside me, unable to escape until I thrashed and yelled and cried and let it drip out of my pores, this energy has me bound and gagged. It is separate, an outside force pinning me to the ground and insisting I pay attention.

I choose to stop fighting, to let it be. To let *them* speak.

I close my eyes and I am in a desert, the same desert that came to me on the day I saw bloodshed in the streets, when I fell into my bed and the sheets turned to sand and I shoveled handfuls of it into my mouth one after the other. Dusk settles on the barren landscape, this time dotted only by small, controlled fires and people milling about between the flames and their tents. In the middle of the settlement is a large post, staked in the dirt looming high above the gray flatlands. A dark creature hangs from the wood, its black wings bound and bolted to the horizontal beams. It is conscious, but immobile. Helpless. Numb. The people know it is there, but they do not pay attention.

The creature's crimson eyes flutter open. It looks at me as it jerks to loosen the cross's hold.

"Help us. Set us free."

What happened to you?

"We don't belong here but we all got caught."

Who are you?

"We are anyone who died here and didn't get out."

How many are you?

"We are countless. The air is so muggy, so heavy with us."

Why are you here?

"Why not? Darkness prevails some places. In others, it cannot. Here it can. So stand back."

I'm so sorry you're trapped.

"You can't will us to die."

The creature flails and bangs its body on the trunk of the post and comes crashing back onto it with an unforgiving thunk. Blood drips from its beak and wings, matting the feathers together with deep, red thread. It cannot escape and it is suffering and the people know it's there, but they do not pay attention.

"This was our destiny the whole time."

I'm so sorry you're afraid to be free.

"Not even God could set us free."

I'm so sorry you have to suffer something worse than death.

"Leave it or you'll suffer too."

The creature twists itself upside down, head toward the ground, front of the body facing the cross, wings wrung and dripping with blood like a twisted, dirtied handkerchief. It uses its talons to push away from the wood in one last attempt to rip itself away. The beam shakes and the desert beneath it cracks and loosens just enough for a moment of hope. It pushes against the beam harder and harder, thrashing as the people mingle around without giving the creature a second glance. It exhausts itself in the fight and falls limp. It knows it will die here. It knows it will never break free. It will bleed to death.

I run through the people and past the burning fires, my arms outstretched as I near the post. I bury my fingers into the creature's wings, searching for the metal spikes lodged into its flesh. Its wings are large and twisted, thick with drying blood. I can't find where the wounds end and the spikes begin. The creature twitches and gasps for air.

"It was hopeless to struggle the whole time."

I'm so sorry you couldn't free your wings and fly.

"It felt safer to keep things the same."

I'm so sorry you couldn't trust life anymore.

"It would have taken a miracle."

I'm so sorry you gave up just at the wrong moment.

"The miracle never came".

I'm so sorry you didn't realize how close you were to freedom.

The creature takes one last gasp and lets it out with a final thump. I feel the fight leave its wings and it hangs limp from the beams. I look around at the people. A few of them make eye contact, but then they look away and turn back to stoke their fires and tend to their roasting meat. I dig through the creature's feathers, peeling the dried blood off its skin until I find the spikes. Each one is just a few inches long, no wider than a pencil. How could such a small piece of metal thwart this magnificent flight? I pluck out bloodied feathers to get a better look. The spikes are barely attached to the creature's flesh. Just a few more pulls and it would have been free. But the struggle took its toll. Even if it had released itself from the binds, the damage to its wings would have been too much.

With a gentle tug I free its left wing and then the right. The creature falls to the ground in a clump. I bring myself to the ground and lie next to it, our heads inches apart in the bloodied dirt.

I'm so sorry you knew you were going to die and there was nothing you could do to stop it.

I listen for an answer but only the breeze responds.

The wind picks up and I choke on the dust and decay. I try to cough to release it, but it is stuck in me and it needs to get out. I open my mouth as wide as it will go and cough into the carpet until my throat burns and I can take a full breath.

Maybe this is it, I think. *Maybe this is how I finally, officially lose it. Someone will walk in and witness me curled up on the floor, sweaty and still swollen with purple limbs, and they will call for help.* But in my heart I know no one will come. If they did, they wouldn't believe me when I say I am infected by this room, pinned to this floor, and trapped by everything that came before me. They wouldn't believe me when I say maybe this is what happens to those who are left behind. Dying is easy. Living in the shadows of the dead is hard. They would put me back on drugs and send me home because they wouldn't understand that feeling this is better than feeling nothing at all. They wouldn't understand that maybe, just maybe, what I'm hearing and seeing in my mind's eye isn't the mental reel of a madwoman, but of a vital force tuning into another frequency, remembering the facets of human suffering that came before. Maybe that's all depression is. A kind of remembering without the tools to release the memories.

At least now I am no longer scared. I know this part of me exists. I know I wasn't so much born with it as much as I was born of it, this remembering etched not only into me, but into the tender soul of every human who ever was and ever will be. I know the deepest cavern of my mind is filled with the horror and pain and sorrow of everything that came before me. It is filled with those killed at the hands of others, in quantities big and small, over the past hundreds of thousands of years, in places I've walked upon and places I will never go. It is populated with everyone destined to wander the street starving but hopeful, and with those who sit atop the throne, fat and bewildered by their own power.

It is the random assortment of people stuffed next to me in each of the metal bullets of planes, trains, and busses over the years, our fates blindly wrapped in the trust of a single soul in the driver's seat. It is the myriad of others who screwed the screws and forged the steel and discovered the flow of electricity from a bright gap in the dark sky to a small key dangling off a kite.

It is the creatures who roamed this Earth. It is the gods who settled their fate. It is the trees and the land, burning to the south. It is the broken promises of mortal men. It is my father and his anger living in the walls of our house like the mold scattered in the corners of this room. It is the war he fought and the people he hurt and the people who hurt him. It is the daughter he fathered and the woman he loved and the people who loved him.

It is him. And me. Us. It is us.

～～～～～～～～

I come to and peel myself off the Kuala Lumpur carpet. I call Alan in a panic, worried I am marching ever closer to what looks like a full-on breakdown. But this is something bigger. I feel it. This is a job for Alan and spiritual alchemy, not for Kathy the psychologist, not for a few little pills, not for my mother. My mother doesn't need this burden. She will take it on. But Alan can help me transmute this, whatever it is, I hope.

When I finally get him on the phone, I pace from corner to corner in my apartment, looking for a spot to huddle where the Wi-Fi can hold our call without gurgling our voices. Eventually I discover the signal in my bathroom is the strongest, so I crawl into my empty bathtub and put Alan on speakerphone. I tell him about the creature with crimson eyes. I tell him I need help. I don't know what's happening, but we need to stop whatever it is, stop whatever they are.

Alan gets to work on compassion statements, and I close my eyes and repeat. But *they* don't stop. With each "I'm so sorry" the images in my mind get stronger, flushing me with visions of destruction pieced together not only from my own lifetime of experiences, but of places I've never been and war I've never fought. The images come at me like lemmings falling off a cliff.

I am a little girl wandering through Dresden's smoking rubble, covering her ears in anticipation of the sounds of combat.

"I'm so sorry whichever way you go, you're lost."

There's no good and right direction.

"I'm so sorry there's no way out of this place."

I am lost in a desert.

"I'm so sorry there wasn't any water anywhere."

There wasn't any life anywhere.

"I'm so sorry you knew what was coming but you couldn't do anything about it."

I am a man covered with burns.

"I'm so sorry no one wanted you that way."

I don't know how to get revenge.

"I'm so sorry they broke your heart."

I am a little girl, trapped in a cage and forced to perform for her food.

"I'm so sorry you had to make them laugh to eat."

You are the entertainment.

"I'm so sorry you got lost in the character."

I am a little boy, fallen overboard off a wooden canoe and drowning in the Indian Ocean.

"I'm so sorry it's so hard to breathe."

No one can rescue you.

"I know this is all coming up for you and it's hard," Alan says, taking a break from the statements, "but I'm glad you got off the medications."

I push my legs and back into the bathtub and feel the weight of the porcelain underneath me.

"Before, when you were on the meds," Alan continues, "people basically said, 'Let's push all that down and let's medicate it.' You were getting pushed out of your own self, in suspended animation, halfway between the soul world and barely in your body. But I believe this is happening because whether you know it or not, you have the ability to integrate back in."

"Alan, I want to believe you, but that's hard to do given that I'm in Kuala Lumpur and I don't want to go outside because it's too fucking loud, so I'm holed up in a bathtub and repeating phrases to a man I've never met because I'm talking to bird ghosts in my head."

He bursts out laughing. "Oh that's funny. I mean it's terrible, I know, but it's also really funny."

He keeps laughing into the phone. His delighted chortle becomes contagious and, after a few seconds of feeling sorry for myself, I realize Alan is right. This whole situation, at a quick glance, is ridiculous. I start laughing too. I start laughing so hard my eyes well up with a different kind of tears. To anyone else this would all seem so crazy. Nine months ago I was functioning at a state just a few rungs higher than anaesthetized. That, somehow, fell on the spectrum of "normal." Then I stopped taking all the drugs and my brain went KABOOM, but now I care that I am alive and I don't want to die and now I'm scared of dying and I want a future. I want the present.

Maybe it's not about coming back to who I was before I was medicated. I can't go back before my father died, to the body and mind I knew through the eyes of a child. I am not a child. I am a grown-ass woman who also happens to be crying in a dirty bathtub because sometimes thoughts get dark and sometimes the mind runs wild and sometimes the solution is not instant and there is no app to download, no filter to swipe, no pill to swallow that can erase the fact that this is human. That I am human. That maybe it will take longer than five and a half months to equalize after a decade and a half of experiencing life through the warped lens of antidepressants. Maybe I tore it all down, and with Alan I'm clearing the rubble. Maybe the crimson-eyed creature was the last boulder to move. Maybe now it's time to rebuild.

Alan and I settle down, the stale air filtered by the lightness of laughter.

"So what do I do about this?" I ask, looking for actionable ways to move forward. "I need to be able to, you know, function."

"Well, maybe we start by accepting that this is just part of who you are. You're super-sensitive to sound and energy. You didn't used to be, but that's because you were medicated. Now you're off them, and you know who you are a bit more. So maybe instead of trying to make where you are more tolerable, take control and find a more tolerable place. A place that works better for you. What do you think? Can you get out of Kuala Lumpur?"

16

I pack a bag. I find a bus. It takes me to Sekinchan.

I am searching for open sky. I want to be able to look out over the land and see nothing but earth—not a skyscraper, construction crane, or hurried soul. I want to find a pocket of this country that I love, to be able to leave Malaysia with a memory of peace, not chaos. I want to walk onto the street without running into another Remote, without having to share an experience. I want to go where I cannot be found. To where I can be less space.

I have three days. In three days I need to be back on a bus to Kuala Lumpur so I can pack up and go with the rest of the group to Thailand. We have a schedule to keep. Month One of Remote Year is almost over, and I still don't know everyone's names. That's a problem for another day. Today, I am alone.

Gone are the days where solo travel is a bumbling adventure into the unknown. Even the most remote places in the world have been explored by Google, so when the bus driver blows past my stop and drops me three miles away from where I'm going, all I have to do is check my phone, turn around, and hoof it. Still, it is well over 100 degrees and the sun beats down as if it is shining just for me. The air is thick with humidity, but out here in the countryside, the horizon is clear. The strata have no interest in wide fields of rice, and the only thing hanging in the air are white egrets soaring over the paddies.

I take my first deep breath in weeks.

I stop at a roadside restaurant to ask for water. A man lies on a mattress off to the side of a dark room, surrounded by empty tables and plastic chairs. This is his home and his business. Today, apparently, business is slow. I point at my empty water bottle, hoping for a refill or a cold bottle. The man goes to his cooler, grabs a can of Coke, pours it into a plastic bag, and knots it with a straw sticking out the top. I take the bag and shrug, too hot to bother getting lost in translation. I give the man a few crumpled ringgits, nod my head in thanks, and turn away.

Already soaked in sweat, I take a sip of my Coke and walk. The sweet bubbles don't quench my thirst, but they cool my throat. I find a dusty path that leads through the rice fields and in the general direction of my guesthouse. The wind picks up and rustles the grassy shoots rising from the rice paddy's floodwater, rippling the landscape like a pebble dropped into a still pond. In the distance, a single figure tends to the rice. Beyond the figure, I can see my destination: a small collection of rainbow-painted shipping containers converted into a humble homestay.

The path is made of fine dirt, sun-bleached the color of bone. With each step my flip-flops kick up a cloud of dust that clings to my sweaty skin. I try to cool myself by thinking of the first evening snow in New York, when it blankets the city in peaceful, frigid fluff. Every year I'd put on my boots, wrap Buffy in her pink sweater, and walk. The city was quiet then. Only the two of us were ever out, the streets calm for just one night while everyone else warmed themselves behind closed doors and the city scrambled to oil up last year's snowblowers. With the quiet came a citywide sense of relief, as if New York spent all year waiting, begging for the first night of snow so it could finally rest.

The bright-pink-and-yellow shipping containers emerge against the fields of green, but still I have a ways to go. I try to keep my focus on winter New York nights to distract myself from the oppressive heat, but sweat is pouring out from every pore in my body and I feel like I am sticking to the muggy, soupy air. My father pops into my head, scratching himself with a wrench in his garage on a hot Nevada day.

"Butt rash," he grunts, and returns to tightening a bolt. I laugh at the memory, glad to have my father turn up and keep me company on the long walk.

When I arrive at the hostel, drenched and caked with dust, the owner, Wilson, is behind a small reception desk. His face drops at the sight of me. He pushes his chair away with a screech and leaves the room, slamming a sliding-glass door shut behind him. I stand in the lobby, confused, until he returns a few minutes later with an armful of ice-cold bottles of water.

"Here!" he says to me, frantically unscrewing the caps. "I expected you many hour ago. I thought you were not coming! Where did you come from? Are you hungry? Drink!"

I down a bottle of water in one long gulp and ask for another. When I can feel my tongue again, all I can say is, "Can I take a shower?"

"Yes! Come, follow me. You like yellow? I put you in the yellow room. But you are the only guest tonight so you can stay in whatever color you like!" Wilson scuttles about the office with the pep of a cartoon mouse, a perky smile plastered on his bespectacled face while he gathers my room key and tidies up the office.

"Yellow is my favorite color," I tell him as he leads me to a canary-yellow shipping container with a single bed, small desk, and a row of windows overlooking the rice paddy. The room is freshly painted, bright with crisp, white linens, yellow pillows, and paintings of pink-and-purple birds. Every corner of the room bursts with joy. I don't want to dirty it, so I drop my bag in the corner and go straight into the lukewarm shower, fully clothed. Dirt falls off of me in clumps and leaves a layer of mud on the bathroom floor. This is a Malaysian bathroom, though, and they are always wet. They all come with a little water pistol called a "bum gun" used exclusively for . . . well, rinsing your bum. Consequently, Malaysian bathrooms are watertight, the floors pitching down to a drain. So I take the bum gun and hose off the entire room, rinsing the filth away. When I step out of the bathroom, a wave of air conditioning hits me. I stand there and let the cold air chill me, naked and finally clean.

I dress and go back to the reception desk. Wilson pops to attention.

"Better?" he asks.

"So much better, thank you. The bus driver dropped me off on the other side of town, so I had to walk here."

"You must be tired, and hungry!"

"Tired, no. Hungry, yes. I'm told I should find some shrimp."

"You want local food?" Wilson asks, perplexed.

"Yes. Whatever you recommend."

Wilson wipes a smudge off his glasses, thinking for a moment before saying, "Good local restaurants very hard for foreigners to find. I go out and bring you something?"

I shake my head. "I'd like to go somewhere, see a bit of the town."

Wilson goes quiet and thinks. I get the impression he spends much of his time alone in this sleepy town, in his sleepy hostel. It seems we are both destined for a meal alone, so I ask him if he would like to join me for dinner.

Wilson lights up at the suggestion.

"Wherever you recommend," I tell him. "Dinner's on me."

"Okay! Let us go!"

Wilson scurries me out the front door and locks it behind me. He takes me to his car, a clunky, beat-up, gray Honda hatchback, and leads me to the passenger's seat on the left side. He opens the door for me and I settle in as he catches the eye of one of his employees milling about on the grounds.

"Just one minute, so sorry. I see my contractor. I need to tell him something." Wilson closes the door and scampers off. While I wait for him, I think of the last yellow cab ride I took as a New York City resident. In the wee hours of the morning, just two months ago, I loaded my suitcase into the trunk and climbed in, one final bagel and lox cradled under my arm. As we drove away from my building and toward the airport, it was like an invisible thread emerged from my shoulder blades and anchored itself back in my apartment. The thread unraveled and tightened with distance, reminding me that no matter how far I travelled, I was still connected to the woman who lived in that space, with the window beckoning her to come through. Sitting in Wilson's car here in Sekinchan, the invisible thread aches between my shoulder blades. No one knows where or who I am. No one can find me if I need to be found. Yet I am calm here among the rice, and the thread feels like it's reaching the end of its length.

Wilson returns to the car and begins driving toward the sea. The thread pulls tighter with each kilometer, wearing thin as he turns a corner and heads into a neighborhood.

The smell of sunbaked fish and motor oil hits me before I see the water. We stop in front of Lee Chuan Fishery, a stilted structure standing thanks to a little sheet metal and a lot of prayer.

"But can you take the Malaysian food?" Wilson says over the idling car motor, worried. "Is it too much for a foreigner's stomach? I think many foreigners cannot take our food."

"I'll be fine," I tell him. "I promise. This is what I came for."

Wilson leads me through the unmarked entrance and we emerge on the docks, greeted by rusted fishing boats and tanks of wiggling fish and crawling crustaceans. Lee Chuan sits on a sunken couch in the corner, shirtless and puffing a cigarette. He acknowledges our presence with a grunt and a wave in the direction of his morning catch. Wilson and I go to work pointing at what will become our dinner: half a dozen oysters, a few mantis prawns, jumbo shrimp, some sort of flat fish—all to be given just a flash of heat before being served alongside citrus and hot sauce.

We sit on the dock and crack open a large Tiger beer—a treat for Wilson, a Chinese descendant living in a Muslim country. Sharia Law forbids Muslims from consuming or selling alcohol, so finding a stiff drink in Malaysia is tricky and expensive. Malaysia has one of the highest alcohol taxes in the world, which drives the cost of a drink up into the realm of New York or London prices. This one beer costs about the same as one night in Wilson's hostel, but I don't care. This night is about freedom and company and quiet. When we finish one beer, we order a second to wash down the piles of seafood arriving one after the other. Wilson and I talk, not about anything in particular. He asks me about New York. I ask him about Malaysia. We speak slowly because although Wilson understands English, he is not fluent. We laugh over translation errors, like how when I ask for "milk" in a café, I get a can of condensed milk. I have to ask for "fresh milk" Wilson tells me, to get what comes from a cow.

I ask him about his business, and he tells me he used to work for his family's antique store, but he wanted something of his own. It's only been a few weeks since he opened, and I am the first Western person to book a room.

"Do you like it?" he asks with concerned, hopeful eyes. "Will people like you like it? I wonder if anyone will." Wilson looks away from me and out toward the sea, mulling over the decisions that led him here. I don't know how to tell this strange man, my new friend, that his colorful shipping containers on top of a rice paddy are part of the antidote I've been searching for. I don't yet have the language for what it means to feel steady, even if it's just over dinner. Here, across the table from Wilson with Lee Chuan frying up a fresh-caught fish behind me, I feel a sureness in myself, in my choices. I don't know what this year will bring, but I am beginning to think if yesterday I was on the floor of my Kuala Lumpur apartment and today I've turned it around enough to enjoy a meal with a kind stranger, then maybe, just maybe, I will be okay. So I raise my glass of beer to him and look him in the eye.

"It's perfect," I tell him. "Thank you for creating it."

Our glasses clink and we take a sip. Lee Chuan comes to clear our plates as the sun falls behind a row of fishing boats.

"The fireflies will be out tonight," Wilson says, looking to the sky. "Would you like to see them?"

I nod, feeling the faint twinge of the invisible thread trying to pull me back. But here in Sekinchan, there isn't anywhere else to be. No deadlines to meet. No one to impress. It is just me, my new friend, and the sea.

~~~~~~~~~

I spend the night with the fireflies and do nothing the next morning except write and sip instant cappuccinos in a hot-pink shipping container Wilson transformed into a café. Bare Edison bulbs hang from the ceiling and reflect off windows overlooking the rice paddy, giving the brilliant-green landscape an air of golden sparkle. I write without earplugs, without headphones, the words in my head singing loud while the paddy hums.

When my stomach rumbles I find Wilson in the blue shipping container, tending to the books at reception, beads of sweat glistening on his brow.

"Hello! How are you? Did you sleep okay? Was the bed comfortable? I don't know if the bed is comfortable because it is new and not many people sleep in it. Do you need anything? Is the air-con cold enough? Sekinchan very hot today."

Wilson takes a short breath and tugs at the collar of his T-shirt.

"You look like you need a nap and some air-con," I say.

Wilson laughs. "Yes. But so much to do! Can I get anything for you?"

"I'm looking for some lunch." I point to a pile of ramshackle bicycles in the corner. "Can I take one of those into town?"

Wilson's eyes widen and he gives me the same concerned look from yesterday. "You want to take bicycle into town by yourself? It is very hot!"

"I know, it's okay. It's not far."

"Okay! Yes!" Wilson scurries to the bikes and lines them up, their rusty kickstands barely holding the bikes' weight. He checks the tires; most are flat. He checks the seats; most are rusted. He runs to a toolbox, grabs a hammer, then turns a bike with half-filled tires on its side and whacks at the seat until it dislodges from its rusty hold. He flips the bike over, tightens a screw.

"Your chariot, Miss Brock!" I like the way Wilson mispronounces my name and when he hands me the bike I am smiling, light for the first time since arriving in Malaysia. Wilson was right. It is hot as hell out here, but when I get on the bike and start pedaling down the dirt road toward town, the air cools as it rushes past me.

In town, I find an outdoor market and order a plate of *nasi lemak* from a woman wearing a hijab. She smiles at me, looks curious. I am wearing shorts and a T-shirt. She's covered head to toe. When I pull a wad of ringgits out of my bra, the woman turns bright-red and struggles to contain her giggles. She calls over another woman who is spooning piles of coconut rice onto plates, points to me, then mimes how I pulled the cash out of my bosom. I get my change and they both watch me with giddy eyes and roar with laughter when I place the change back in my bra. I smile, stand back, look my bare self up and down.

"Where else am I supposed to put it?" I shrug, laughing too. I don't know if the two women can understand my words, but they understand what I'm trying to say. Feminine secrets are the same in every language. The two women cackle with delight.

I get my plate of *nasi lemak,* a national staple of coconut rice covered in sweet and spicy sambal, crispy anchovies, peanuts, and a fried egg. When I sit down to eat it, I am joined by a stray dog who waits for dropped morsels. She doesn't seem to bother with the locals. She must know I'm an easy target. For every two bites I take, I toss one in the dirt. When I get up to leave, the pup follows me and runs alongside the bike until I hit the edge of town.

I pedal down the dirt road leading out of town and take a left into the rice paddies. I continue down the long, straight roads cutting through the green field, racing into the horizon. With each push I get further from Kuala Lumpur, further from New York City, further from the past five months, further from the past fifteen years. The invisible thread hooked to my shoulder blades tightens, frays, just barely holds on.

"More of this," I whisper, almost begging the oncoming wind.

More of this peace, this freedom, this space.

I pedal. Into the horizon. Into infinite space. I pedal as the sky turns gray and the temperature drops. I pedal as the rain falls. I pedal as the little drops hit my skin and I can feel their edges, but this time they are not bullets—they are soft. They hit my bare arms with a tender patter and rinse the dust, sweat, and ick of Kuala Lumpur, of New York. I pedal as the rain fills my eyes and

I close them, shake my head, and in one blink, when I open up my eyes, the world seems saturated with color.

This is relief. Relief from the heat. Relief from the beating sun. Relief from the pressure. With each pedal, relief.

I pedal until lightning strikes the horizon, followed by a boom of thunder and immediate sheet of rain. I stop and let the bike fall to the ground. Another snake of light slithers across the sky, and in the sudden burst of light, I feel the frayed thread finally break free. It falls from between my shoulder blades and dissolves into the earth, taking with it all remaining connection to the woman I was. The person who emerged out of the past fifteen years and just two days ago was shattered on the Kuala Lumpur floor, she doesn't exist in this place. I know in my gut that right now I am safe from outside forces. More important though, in this solitude, in this anonymity, in this moment, I feel safe from myself.

I open my mouth and take a drink. The fat droplets moisten my tongue. *More of this.*

The droplets hit harder. Come quicker. The rain falls in sheets, sideways and frontways and backways, pounding me from all angles until I am soaked down to the ringgits in my bra. I open my arms wide and let the rain come. I stand. Sway. Hold onto the relief for seconds, minutes, I don't know how long, it doesn't matter. I hold onto the relief until from somewhere within me I hear *"it is time to go back"* and I pedal.

I pedal to my temporary home. To my temporary friend. To my temporary life. Tomorrow I go back to Kuala Lumpur. And the day after that, Thailand.

For now there is nothing left to do but ride in the rain. I pedal. And beg. *More of this.*

17

We arrive on the island of Koh Phangan, Thailand just after dusk. A scrawny, middle-aged man stands out in the bustle of my cranky travel companions, all of whom are scrambling about the ferry to gather up scattered pieces of their lives. The man is still and stern. He looks like the sort that mothers feared their daughter would bring home for dinner—the good-for-nothing punk who passed the time by lighting things on fire and stealing booze. I imagine the man had hair back then, probably. A little meat on his bones, perhaps. But now, bald with gray scruff and a face full of piercings, he seems too slim for his tattooed skin, and it hangs off his frame like one of Dali's clocks. He and I stare at each other for a moment. He adjusts his backpack, folds his inked arms across his chest, and looks away. I step off the ferry and adjust to the salty air. The thin man passes in front of me and disappears into the night.

In the dark, I fumble for my bags and load them into Koh Phangan's version of a taxi, which is really more of a pickup truck with two shaky benches half-bolted to the truck bed. A dozen of us squeeze in shoulder to shoulder, our knees and elbows sticking to each other as we jostle down the main road. We pull out of town and head to our Remote Year accommodations, bungalows on the beach about twenty minutes north. The road to our new homes is long and desolate, or so it seems in the darkness. An occasional streetlight pops up, the orange tint illuminating our sweaty limbs all tangled together like a pile of twigs resting in the glow of a campfire. No one speaks.

We come to a near halt and turn down a narrow dirt road. Palm trees sweep against the truck and prickle our backs through the bed's metal cage.

Deep, croaking groans from frogs and monitor lizards emerge from the bush, both welcoming us to our new home and warning us that we are trespassing on their territory. The taxi stops in the middle of a makeshift parking lot. We file out of the truck, grab our things, and hoof through the sand to get to our bungalows. I fiddle with the padlock barely securing a damp, wooden door to the crème-de-menthe-colored structure and push the creaky door open, bringing a wave of sand with me. Something furry scampers through my legs and runs to the other side of my one-room bungalow.

I switch on the light and am greeted by an orange kitten, no bigger than a handful, meowing at me and brushing her long tail through the dust on the floor. I drop my bags and crouch toward her, my heart bursting with joy to be greeted by a fuzzy, little creature.

"Hi, sweetheart!" I scoop her up in my hands and she blinks at me with big, green eyes. I can feel her ribs through her downy folds, but otherwise she seems to be in good shape. She isn't mangy or full of ticks and seems clean for a beach cat.

"What's your name?" I ask her, half expecting her to respond as I bring her to my chest and rock her like a baby. "Madeline? Or maybe Matilda? I like Matilda." I grab her underneath her front legs and hold her out in front of me. "Hey, Matilda! It's nice to meet you."

I put Matilda down and look at my home for the month. Though the bungalow looks secure-ish from the outside, inside it is a different story. The walls are made of bamboo and don't connect to the thatched roof, leaving a few inches of space that open to the outside. The bathroom is more like an outhouse, tacked onto the already-shoddy structure and only half covered by the roof. The showerhead hangs over the toilet, and a few dead roaches lie belly up in the corner. The kitchen is nothing more than a single induction burner and a sink, with a perpetually humming refrigerator. I open it up and stick my head in, breathing in the cool, stale air.

Something thunks and hisses across the bungalow and I turn to see Matilda hunting a cockroach in the corner, bashing her little body into the wall as she corners the roach. She hits the vile insect with her paw until the thing stops moving, gives it a sniff, and then eats it in one bite. I pick her up and put her outside for the night, figuring I don't have a litter box. Not that she knows about the particulars of a litter box. The entire island is her litter box.

I wake up the next morning to the faint sound of the ocean and Matilda meowing outside my door. I open the door and she darts in, leaping from the nightstand to the bed to the floor, eventually settling on her back and pawing at the edge of the mosquito net. This is her home, clearly. I am simply renting a room.

I check my email and see a message from Alan telling me that Hurricane Matthew is ravaging Haiti with 140-mile-per-hour winds, prompting Florida to begin emergency evacuation procedures. He says he will reach back out when it's safe to go home, but I know that if the damage is bad, it could be weeks before he and I speak again.

I watch Matilda tangling herself in the mosquito net, trying to process the realization that I am on my own. I don't know if I am ready yet. Maybe it's too soon. Malaysia almost broke me. Thailand might too.

A breeze shakes my thatched roof, sending a whiff of salty air into my bungalow and reminding me I'm mere steps from the sea. I push open the warped, creaky door and the brilliant, sparkling ocean, once hidden in the night, now reveals itself before me. The water is calm, little two-inch waves breathing up and down over the sand. Palm trees dot the beach like mushrooms on a forest log, seeming to pop up here and there with no particular order. The beach is alive, filled with scuttling sand crabs, crisscrossing from one hole to another. A brown-and-white dog amuses herself by chasing the crabs into their tunnels and then digging them out, flinging the poor crustaceans across the sand.

I slip on my shoes, still wearing my shorts and tank top from the night before, and wander toward the turquoise water. A forty-five-foot long, double-mast sailboat sits capsized in the distance, lodged sideways in the coral. The ocean circles it with changing hues of emerald and turquoise, unfazed by the steadfast resident. Somewhere behind me, the door to another Remote's bungalow slams shut. I turn around to see Ross, who I haven't talked to much since orientation, stretching the morning kinks out of his beanpole of a body.

He waves.

I smile back and he goes inside his bungalow.

In the distance, a power saw revs up and my heart drops into my belly. The landscape is different, but the situation is the same.

"Fuck." I sigh and roll my head around my neck, my arms beginning to throb at the first screech.

I look back toward the beached boat and cock my head sideways to right the angle of its mast. The damn ship is a glaring metaphor for my life. Even surrounded by beauty, I am still stuck with myself.

I close my eyes, feel the sun beat down on my skin, and wonder what to do. The peace of Sekinchan still with me, I had hoped that this tropical island would be still, the soothing beach photos littering the internet delivering the same sort of tranquility in person that they exude on the screen. But paradise is loud and I am island-bound for five weeks straight. I can't escape to the countryside like I did in Kuala Lumpur. Koh Phangan is only forty-eight square miles and doesn't even have a postal service. The entire island is the countryside. I am already here.

I am going to have to find an outlet, a pocket of tranquility and space. I refuse to spend this month barricaded in my bungalow, ears submerged in rusty bathwater, in a failed attempt to protect myself from whatever triggers me. That didn't work in Kuala Lumpur and I have no reason to believe it will work in Thailand. I need to learn. I need to adjust. I need to get to know myself in this new body, this new mind.

Alan's soothing voice runs through my mind. *"Maybe we start by accepting that this is just part of who you are."*

Matilda comes bounding out of the bungalow, circles me. I wonder how many cats I would need to offset the number of bugs in my bungalow and then remember how I once entertained the idea of getting a lizard in New York City to eat all the roaches in my apartment.

Matilda flops on her back, showers my feet with sand, then scampers up a palm tree.

The power tool whirs and waves trickle over the beach. I slip off my shoes, stare into the horizon, and dive headfirst into the sea.

~~~~~~~~~~~~

My arms are numb and my heart is pounding as I wait for my ride to the dive resort for my first day of open water scuba certification. I decide to get certified after overhearing a few Remotes—Mike, Val, and Mat—talking about diving. If there is any hope for quiet, it's under the sea. There are no chop saws in the ocean, so I butt into the conversation and ask if I can join.

I have been scuba diving once before, when my mother took me on a vacation to Maui when I was nineteen. There is a photo of me somewhere, a dozen feet under the surface, with a sea turtle paddling along next to me. That's all I remember. That and what it felt like to breathe through the scuba gear in the hotel's crystal-clear pool. The ability to dart back and forth from one end of the pool to another, the cool water rushing over my bare skin with nothing but the sound of my own breath filling my ears, felt like a superpower created just for me. When I popped out of the pool and walked over to my mother, sunning on a lounge chair, she shook her head and said, "You've always been so fearless. I don't know where you get it from."

I shrugged. At the time, I didn't know either.

Now I understand that I was never truly fearless. Wanting the nothingness of death does not a fearless person make. Fearlessness is to be bold, to be courageous in the presence of danger. I was nothing but a drugged-up common coward, too prideful to admit my "fearlessness" was more about the tantalizing power of indifference. I walked to the edge of Earth and dangled my toes over cliffs, and dreamed of turbulence strong enough to send the plane plunging down. I inched my car close to the highway median to see if I felt any different, to see if I felt anything. And when I peered over the cliff's edge or slammed my foot onto the gas, it wasn't that my body didn't feel. My throat thickened and my stomach gurgled and my fingers tingled with anticipation. My physical body felt the threat of danger. But in my mind, nothing registered. I observed the physical signals in my body with the detachment of a soldier in shock, unaware that the mangled limb belongs to him.

But waiting for Mike to pick me up and take me to the dive shop, I am not fearless. I am scared shitless. Not only am I about to strap a thirty-pound canister of steel to my back in order to sink to the bottom of the ocean just to look at fish, but getting to the dive shop requires a ride on the back of Mike's rental motorbike, his death machine. The island is hilly and the roads aren't maintained. Gravel causes inexperienced riders to skid out on tight turns. Stray dogs nap in the middle of the road and coconuts fall from lofty palms, turning an otherwise open road into an obstacle course. But more important, my mother told me I was never, ever allowed to get on a motorcycle. It was her only consistent demand, her only expectation. I could climb Everest, work as a mortician, dress as an alien and insist on being called Dousabella. My mother didn't care how I lived as long as it made me happy and did not include motorcycles. I blame my father. Before I was born, he convinced my mother to go for a little ride around the neighborhood. After he took a few laps around the block, he made the bold move to leave the neighborhood and get on the highway, forever scaring the shit out of my mom. As soon as I was old enough to sit up, she made it clear to my father that if he ever put me on one of his motorcycles, she would divorce him. And if the news reported a fatal motorcycle crash, she told me about it to drive her point home. Motorcycles, motorbikes, anything with two wheels and an engine may as well be cyanide. And yet here I am on an island in Thailand, ready to drink the poison down.

I hear the thin rumble of a motorbike whiz around the corner and Mike pulls up next to me.

"You ready for this?" he asks with a smile. He pulls off his helmet, loses his balance, and falls over, just barely catching himself with one foot before the whole bike topples over.

"Are you sure you know what you're doing on that thing?" I ask. "I am not comfortable with motorcycles."

"Don't worry about it. I practiced yesterday!" Mike is a twenty-seven-year-old software engineer with the naive confidence of a golden retriever puppy thrust into a pack of wolves.

"Go slow," I beg. "Like really slow. As slow as you can."

"I will, I promise. Everyone else crashed because they were going too fast, so I only go as fast as I need to. Here, take my helmet."

Mike tosses me the helmet, but it is too big and the ribboned clasp is broken, so I tighten it with a double knot under my chin, roll my eyes toward the sky, and mutter at my father, "You better keep us safe."

Mike climbs back on the bike and I get behind him.

"Slow," I say one more time, wrapping my arms around his waist.

We putt toward the dive resort, picking up speed in order to get up the hills. I squeeze my arms tight around Mike and hold my breath as the wind rushes by, forcing myself to focus on the views opening wide across the white sand beaches with palm trees lining the coast of Koh Phangan. The jewel-hued water seems to go on for eternity, palm trunks perched on the pure white coast while palm leaves brush against a cloudless sky.

"Holy shit! Look at that!" Mike yells as we hit a summit and the scope of Koh Phangan's beauty reveals itself to us. His words hit the wind and come rushing back at me.

"Eyes on the road!" I yell back, but my response is no match for the draft and Mike just yells "what?" and keeps staring at the horizon.

I clench my legs around the bike, mumbling "keep us safe" all the way until we pull into the dive shop with a thud. I get off the bike as quickly as I can and feel my weight on the ground beneath me.

Mat and Val are waiting. Val is a blond Russian bombshell with an accent right out of a Boris and Natasha cartoon, and Mat is a Polish digital designer whose clientele is primarily sourced from Burning Man VIP tents. Standing next to their motorbike, helmets dangling from their hands, they look like an Eastern European power couple on their way to a photo shoot.

"Did you two get lost?" Mat jokes.

"Har har," I say.

"You look like you need some vodka," Val says.

"Wouldn't hurt," I say, following her into the dive shop, shaky on my legs.

"Well 'ello there, mates." A small, thin Brit takes a long drag from his cigarette. He looks familiar, but I can't place him. "Welcome! I'm Martin."

Mike introduces himself, shakes Martin's hand, and bursts out laughing. "Wait, were you on the plane with us from Kuala Lumpur to Surat Thani?"

"On Sunday?" Martin nods. "Yep, I was. Just moved back 'ere from me old dive shop in the Philippines. You're my first dive group back 'ere in KP."

Mat pipes in. "I remember seeing you in customs! That's crazy. I guess it was meant to be."

And now I remember locking eyes with Martin on the ferry.

He says, "Well it's nice to meet the lot of you. I'm excited to have you 'ere. Fancy a coffee?" Martin gestures to a hot-water thermos and a pile of three-in-one instant coffee. We pour the brown powder into paper cups, let the bittersweet mixture dissolve, and settle ourselves on a warped picnic table.

"Unfortunately we won't be divin' today," Martin continues, dropping his pierced, bald head in disappointment. "Since you are all getting your certification, before you dive we have to have you watch a video and do some paperwork. It is so boring. I mean *really* boring. But we have to do it. Any of you been divin' before?"

I raise my hand. "I went in Hawaii once, but I'm not certified."

"A discov'ry dive, right," Martin says, "so you're a lit'le bit familiar. First things first. I need you all to sign this paperwork in case you die on us. Please answer the questions honestly. If you've got a medical condition, don't say you don't have a medical condition because I can't have you having a heart attack on me at the bottom of the fookin' ocean. Aw'right?"

He passes us the forms and a box of pens, and I start filling out the medical questionnaire:

"Are you presently taking prescription medications?"

For the first time in my adult life, I get to write "no" in bold letters. I feel a twinge of something like pride swell within me. *I did it. Not with much grace or any dignity and I'm still a mess, but I did it.*

"Frequent or severe attacks of hay fever or allergy?"

I write, "Only when the Nevada sagebrush blooms, and luckily we're in Thailand."

"Any form of lung disease?"

"No."

"Behavioral health, mental, or psychological problems?"

I stop writing and look at Mike, Val, and Mat. I barely know these people. They don't need to know.

So I lie. I lie because no one knows about it. I lie because I don't want to give into it. I lie because I got on the motorbike and got this far. I lie because I got on the damn plane and came this far.

I scribble my signature and pass the paper back to Martin along with an inch-thick stack of Thai baht. Martin gathers our cash and stacks it in front of him like a swashbuckling drug lord.

"Right, mates. What we'll have you all do is watch the video, then you all can have lunch, and after we'll talk about it and go over everything. Tomorrow we'll go to the pool for skills in the mornin', and then we'll head out to Sail Rock for your open-water dives the followin' day. Does that work?"

"We need to work in the afternoon, so that's good," Mike says, gesturing to Mat and Val. They are working US hours, which means they clock in before dinner and work well into the night. I write in the morning, before the day has a chance to burrow itself into my head. I tell Martin I'm free only in the afternoon.

"Aw'right, so I'll take these three in the mornin' and then I'll take you in the afternoon." Martin taps the ash of his cigarette and points its tip at me. "And we'll have loads of fun."

18

"Fookin' idiots." Martin holds up his middle finger to nothing in particular and rolls his eyes as the road suddenly turns from pavement to dirt. "They decide to do work on the road, but instead of takin' it up one section at a time, they tear the whole thing up at once."

We are on our way to a resort on the north end of the island that lets the dive shop use its pool. It's just Martin and me in the truck.

"This is the most dangerous part of today," Martin says with a stone face. "Driving to the pool."

We hit a pothole and I bounce so high off the seat that I'm airborne.

"Sorry, mate. It's going to be like this for the next twen'y kilometers."

"Where are you from?" I yell over the rattle of the old pickup truck and the clang of oxygen tanks slamming into each other in the truck bed.

"Just outside of London, a small town in Essex!" Martin takes his eyes off the road and crosses them while flashing a tobacco-stained smile. "Can't you hear it in me'accent?"

This man is batshit-crazy and endearing. I like him already.

"I hear the Brit. Couldn't place the Essex. How did you end up here?" We hit another bump and I grab onto the dashboard to steady myself.

"My twin brother works at a dive shop in Koh Samui, so that's how I first come here years ago. I left to open up my own dive shop in the Philippines with my girlfriend. I did that for a while, but then we broke up and I didn't want to run the shop by me'self. So I called my brother, and he says to me, 'Martin, come home.' This is my home. Koh Phangan is my home. It always

has been. Not London. Not the Philippines. Here. Thailand. Koh Phangan."
The tattooed man goes silent for a moment before adding, "I do miss doner
kebabs in London, though. But that's it. How are you finding your travels so far?"

I pause, unsure of how to answer.

"It's shit. It's amazing. But it's shit. And amazing."

"Sounds a lot like life," Martin smirks, and we drive down the road in
silence until we turn left toward the resort and park. Stilted bungalows and
dirtied huts sit abandoned all around us. The hum of guests and staff are long
gone, their presence replaced with the faint brush of palms rustling in the
wind. The place is eerie, as if no one had stayed in the resort for years and we
are trespassing on haunted ground.

"Pool's this way, mate."

We each grab our bag of scuba supplies and walk down the fractured
tile steps to a pool so thick and rotting-green it may as well have been a
kale smoothie.

"Looks bloody great, doesn't it? No one's gotten a flesh-eating virus yet,
though." Martin snickers as he drops his bag with a thud on a lounge chair
with missing slats. "But who knows, you could be the first."

I look from Martin to the opaque, greenish-brown pool and back to
Martin again. My only consolation is I know Mike, Mat, and Val survived
the morning in this same pool.

"Lovely," I say, glad I've done this once before in a pool where I could
actually see the bottom.

Martin takes a puff off the cigarette living between the fingers of his left
hand, amused at my disgust. "Aw'right now, put on that wetsuit and let's get
you certified."

We strip down to our bathing suits and put on our wetsuits. Even though
it's over ninety degrees in a tropical country, Martin wears a full-body wetsuit
covering him from knobby ankles to bony wrists. His wetsuit is still dripping from
the morning, and with it zipped up, he looks like a waterlogged praying mantis.

I squeeze into my wetsuit, arms and legs mostly bare. After six weeks in
Asia, my body has softened thanks to buttery roti, curries swimming in coconut
fat, and coffee saturated with sweetened condensed milk. *Be less space*, an old
voice whispers to me as I tuck my flesh into the damp spandex. I close my
eyes. Shake my head. Now is not the time for body-image bullshit. Now is the

time to remember how to jump into the open ocean with a thirty-five-pound weight strapped to my back. Nerves tingle throughout my body and I remind myself: *You've done this before. You're here. You paid for it. Suck it in. Suck it up.*

I zip myself up like a roast held together with twine and plop down on the creaking lounge chair.

"Okay, mate. When you did your discov'ry dive, the dive master did all this for you. But since you're gettin' certified, you need to know how to work the equipment." Martin kneels next to me and starts pointing to the various components of the inflatable vest that will theoretically keep me alive. We practice securing my tank to the buoyancy-compensation device better known as the BCD. We clip and unclip the clasps, pull the cords, and examine the hoses before breathing into the regulator and backup regulator.

"This is Thailand," Martin says, squinting into the regulator mouthpiece. "Always check for spiders."

He gets me suited up and puts on his own gear.

"Now, the most important thing before you dive is the buddy check, right mate? We always have a buddy when we're divin'. Today, you're my buddy. You need to check my gear to make sure it's all working, and I check yours. We do this every time before we dive. Every single time. Got it?"

I nod, trying to hide the nerves bubbling inside me, a layer of bile creeping up the back of my throat.

I am barely capable of managing myself.

"Brilliant," Martin says. "All you have to remember is BWARF. First, we have to check the B, the buoyancy." Martin pushes the button on the inflator hose, fluffing me up like a burnt marshmallow. Then he pulls on the hanging tab and shrivels me back down.

"Weights." He looks for the individual kilo weights strapped around my waist.

"Air." He tests the air pressure in each of my regulators and takes a big breath from each.

"Releases." He tugs at all the clips and straps to make sure they're buckled and secure.

"Final." He scans me from head to toe, checking my mask, compass, and fins.

"BWARF," he says, "Because We Aren't Really Fish. Or Bruce Willis Always Ruins Films. And my personal favorite, Bangkok Women Are Really Fellas. It's true. Lots of surprises in Bangkok. Now you check me."

I go through Martin's buddy check and we waddle over to the pool. With one giant stride I remind myself *you've done this before* and step into the green water. I inflate my BCD to bob to the surface. The water feels slippery against my legs and the pool is unsettlingly warm. I feel heavy and encumbered. Even though I know we're in a pool and the cement floor is somewhere underneath me, I can't see my body in the water, and it feels like I'm bobbing on top of the Mariana Trench.

Martin splashes in behind me and swims over.

"Ready?" he asks.

"I'm nervous," I confess, embarrassed because I've done this before and yet I'm still scared.

"I'll be right here," Martin assures me. "Just take it one skill at a time."

He holds his inflator hose over his head and gestures me to do the same. We deflate our BCDs to sink under the surface. I watch as the world around me disappears one inch at a time until I'm submerged. I can make out Martin's outline a few feet in front of me. He signals me to just sit and breathe.

Instead, I panic. I can't control my buoyancy, so my body turns sideways, and I flail around to right myself. But I am surrounded by murky water and I can't tell what's up or down and I am suddenly aware I am breathing through bottled air that's strapped to my back by one tiny, little clasp and *what if the air runs out and what if there's a leak and what if the tank falls off my back and this equipment is made by humans and humans fuck up all the time and I'm sinking down and I can't see the bubbles and I can't see the surface and I can't slow my breath and—*

A hand grabs the weight belt at my hips.

Martin unclips the belt with one hand and steadies me with the other. He adjusts the weight, clips the belt back on me, and lets go. I float smoothly in the water.

Martin swims in front of me and gestures with his hands, but I don't understand what he's asking and I need to understand and I can't catch a full breath, so I shake my head and inflate my vest and as soon as I break the surface I spit out my regulator and pull up my mask and gasp.

Martin pops up a few seconds later.

"What happened?" I spout out before he has a chance to settle himself. I look into his goggled eyes, hoping the murky pool water hides the tears pooled at the bottom of my mask.

"Just a bit too much weight on you, that's all. Ready to go back down?"

He puts his inflation tube above his head and I shout "wait!" and make him explain what we're doing, again. And again after that. We practice descending, regulator recovery, and frog kicking, and I make Martin come to the surface after each exercise to go over the next one. Whatever confidence I once had as a teenager in Hawaii is gone, replaced by a shaking thirty-year-old scared of a pool.

"You're doing aw'right, I promise," Martin says to me after I ask him to explain the drill for the third time. "It's actually easier in the ocean because the visibility is better. This is shit. Really, shit. Just one more exercise." He adjusts his olive-green mask and demonstrates the exercise and narrates what I'm supposed to do, step by step. "I need you to flood your mask and clear it. First you tip the mask away from your face and let it fill with water. Then you'll tip your head back, press the mask on your forehead, and blow out your nose. The pressure will push out the water. When you've done that, you've got to take your mask off underwater, put it back on, and clear it again. Then you've done it! Got it?"

A rotund, hairy man emerges from somewhere in the resort, wearing nothing but a Speedo and yelling something to someone in Russian. Apparently there are guests in this hotel, and I don't want to make a scene. So I nod at Martin, even though my mind can't comprehend the thought of removing my scuba mask in a murky pool, let alone in the salty sea.

We descend.

Martin goes through the drill slowly as I watch, and when he finishes clearing his mask for the second time, he points at me to go. I tip my mask forward and let the water flow in, but as soon as I feel the water on my nose, I forget to breathe through the regulator and I inhale through my nose and choke. I fasten the mask back onto my face, tilt my head a fraction of a degree, and breathe out enough to clear the mask with a meek blurp, but I'm still choking and now I'm coughing and *what if this happens at 100 feet deep and what if I can't breathe and I forget to equalize and I don't make a safety stop and I get the bends and pop an eardrum and my lungs collapse and why are you putting yourself through this, why are you putting yourself in danger and will you ever go back to being fearless?*

I pull on my emergency inflation cord, shoot to the surface of the pool, and rip off my mask. I suck in short, humid breaths and sob into the green water.

Martin floats over and puts his hands on my shoulders as I shake and he looks in my swollen, teary eyes and says, "You did it! I know it's scary, but you did it!"

"I'm sorry. I don't know why . . . " I look away from him. I feel like a child who has done something wrong, but doesn't know how to fix it. "I've done this before. I don't know why I can't do it now."

"But you did do it! You forgot about breathing through your mouth for a second, but you won't do that again."

"I don't know. Maybe this isn't right for me. If I can't even do it in the pool . . . "

"Mate, listen to me. I've been divin' my entire life and I've taught thousands of people how to do it. Lots of people have trouble with this, and I'm telling you, you're doing fine. The others this morning had some trouble too."

I think of Mat, Val, and Mike and I'm glad they're not here to see this.

"We can spend as much time here as you need to feel comfortable. Let's try it again."

"Okay." I nod and breathe and go under again. I don't want to be the only one who quits.

I manage to fill up the mask with just a touch of water and tip my head back to breathe the water out as quickly as I can. Martin claps and cheers underwater like I just broke an Olympic record. He steadies himself and, in slow motion, takes off his mask, puts it back on, and clears out the water. He gestures at me to do the same. I close my eyes as tight as I can and remove my mask, holding my breath even though I know I'm not supposed to. In the darkness, without the thin veil of plastic and rubber against my skin, my edges disappear in the warm water. I think of the last time I lost my edges on the dirty carpet that held my weight in Kuala Lumpur. I remember the red eyes of the bird-like creature on the cross, how it blinked at me before falling to the ground with its last gasp. I remember losing my edges in humidity and paranoia in the subway station a few months ago, when Thailand was just a fantasy and Martin didn't exist. Back then it was the raindrops and a mangled ironing board bringing me to the edge of who I am. Now it is yet another strange country, with yet another strange man, guiding me to find the borders of my soul.

In the slow, underwater movement, I fumble with my mask in the darkness until it's back on my face and hold it to my forehead to clear it out with one, long exhale. I rest for a moment and take in a fresh breath from the regulator, the sound of my inhale lighting up my edges once again. I listen to the sound I make when I breathe into the regulator. It sounds like *schlooooop, schlooooop. Schlooooop, schlooooop.* I have never before noticed the force of my breath, how each inhalation and exhalation demands life.

I let the experience of diving in Maui dissolve into the murky water, knowing the fearlessness was nothing more than the deadening of antidepressants and the ignorance of youth. Now it's like there is a translation error within me, like the language of my past fifteen years no longer makes sense. I can still translate the basics, the day-to-day. Get up. Brush your teeth. Take out the trash.

Schlooooop, schlooooop. Schlooooop, schlooooop.

Sometimes I can recognize new words, new feelings, like the elation of winning *Chopped* or the swirl of color on a canvas or the rush of relief in the Sekinchan rain. I can gesture when the language begins to fail. I can smile when they smile. Nod when they nod. Watch them operate. Imitate. But I can't seem to translate the experiences of my old life.

If I can't translate all I've known, all I've believed, and all I've understood into the parameters of this unmedicated life, what am I left with? Who am I left with?

***

Mat, Mike, Val, and I load into the dive shop's boat with Martin and a few dive masters. We voyage north to Sail Rock, a large stone in the Gulf of Thailand housing a magical ocean world. Sail Rock announces itself quietly, beginning as a mere grain of sand disturbing an otherwise flat horizon. As the boat pushes forward, the stone grows like a seed in soil, eventually revealing itself as the only unwavering piece of land for miles in any direction. With the open ocean jostling the boat from side to side, we suit up and strap on our gear. All four of us are nervous. Val suggests we take a shot of vodka to calm our nerves. Had she handed me a bottle, I would have gulped it down.

On deck, Martin decides Mat and I will be buddies, and he instructs us to hold hands at the start of the dive so we don't lose each other. We jump off the boat one after the other, landing in the tropical water with a rubber-finned smack. With the panic of yesterday's pool training still fresh in my mind, I fiddle with my mask, worried it will flood and I will have to clear it underwater.

I pull off the mask and spit into it in order to keep it from fogging, then hold it to my face as I peek my head through the water's surface. Just below us lurk thousands of tiny jellyfish.

I spring up. "Martin!"

Martin is adjusting Val's mask a few yards away.

"Martin!" I yell until he looks my way. "Look down!"

He pokes his head under the ocean like a bird looking for worms and comes up a few seconds later, without panic. "I've never seen that before in all me time on KP! They must've floated over with the current after last night's storm. Nothin' to worry about, though."

"Can we still dive?" Mike asks after taking a look himself.

"Of course we still dive! They're harmless li'l things. Just brush 'em off. We'll stay shallow and swim around the rock to see if it clears up. If we see a box jelly, I will bang the hell out of my tank with my rod here"—Martin holds up a metal rod and taps his tank—"and that means you need to pay attention to me and look where I'm pointing. If it's a box jelly, swim the fook away. Ready, mates?" And with that, Martin holds up his inflator hose over his head and descends.

Mat and I look at each other, waiting for the other to make the first move.

"I guess we go down now," Mat says with a shaky laugh, holding up his inflator hose.

I nod, raise my hose. We descend, coming to a halt just a few feet below the surface. Martin gestures for Mat and me to hold hands. I put my hand on top of his, and he squeezes back with an equal amount of fear. At least we are nervous together.

The jellyfish seem to stay put below us, so I look around. I can see the underside of Sail Rock in front of us, adorned with specs of bright-colored fish and coral. I try to relax and steady my breathing as we kick, taking care to balance my buoyancy in the water so I don't lose control like I did in the pool. Suddenly the current changes and my legs dip. The current swells and pushes behind me and, in one oceanic breath, jellyfish surround me. Mat and I look at each other, eyes wide behind our masks. Up ahead, Martin and the others continue on, unfazed. Mat and I squeeze each other's hands a little harder.

Something tickles against my wrist and I look down to see a jellyfish wrapped gently around Mat's and my intertwined palms. I watch it hover for a second, waiting to see what it will do. Then it latches its tentacles onto me, sending a searing pain across the back of my hand. I scream into the regulator; a wall of bubbles surrounds me. Mat and I break our grasp and shake off the jellyfish as Martin kicks over. He examines my hand underwater and, using sign language, asks if I want to continue. I shake my head no, signal to the surface, and ascend. The others pop up around me.

"What happened?" Mike asks as he spits out his regulator.

"Just a lit'le sting, that's all! Hell of a first dive, isn't it, mates?" Martin laughs as he examines my reddening hand. "So what do you all want to do? It will be clear around the other side of the rock."

Mat holds up his stung hand. "It doesn't hurt too bad."

The splotchy sting on my hand changes from pink to rose to red.

"As long as it's safe, I want to keep going," Mike says, his blind confidence both perplexing and encouraging. Mat and Val nod in agreement.

"It is safe," Martin says to all of us. "The jellies sting a lit'le, but they won't kill you." He turns to me, "You good to keep going?"

I don't want to be the one to put an end to the dive, so I agree to keep going. Without me asking, Martin pairs Mat with another dive master and keeps me as his buddy. We descend again and swim together, slowly, while Martin uses his metal rod to move the jellies out of our way, but soon another current comes and we are surrounded again. Martin's long-sleeved, full-length wetsuit protects him from the menacing creatures. My short-sleeved, short-legged suit leaves me exposed. The jellies find my skin and each sting feels like burning iron and soon my uncovered body is on fire with a dozen stings.

I shoot to the surface, in too much pain to keep going. The others continue. Martin comes up behind me, unscathed.

"Let's get you back to the boat," he says as the color leaves my face.

We turn on our backs and kick away from Sail Rock.

I climb onto the bow and the skipper takes one look at me, strips off my gear, pulls off my wetsuit, and douses me in a bucket full of vinegar. The acetic acid cools the stings swelling in bulbous lumps on my arms and legs. Martin asks if I'm okay to let him return to the group. I shoo him away and lay on the deck to let the sun dry off my tender body. Through my haze, I think about the dozens of third-degree burns I weathered while working in kitchens, and how the pain never fazed me. The scars left from those burns remain, but the scar tissue couldn't protect me here. Yet another question I'll never be able to answer: *Is my severe reaction to the stings because this is who I am? Or is it a physiological overcorrection from years of antidepressant numbing, that one day will stabilize?*

I groan at the unknown and nod off to sleep, lightly pickling in the sun.

The group returns from their dive forty minutes later. The water cleared just a minute or so after I turned around, they tell me, leaving them with a stunning, crystalline first dive. Their stings have already faded. Mine are still hot and pulsing. I splash them with another glug of vinegar.

The captain puts out a container of Panang curry and rice, made for us by his wife. The group swarms over the curry, shoveling it in in big mouthfuls in between a ricochet of questions and comments.

"Did you see the big school of round fish when we came around the corner? Martin, what were those?"

"Longfin batfish."

"And all the barracuda!"

"Then there was that real ugly eel."

"Martin, what kind was it?"

"A moray eel."

"What was the yellow polka-dotted one?"

"Yellow boxfish."

"When do we go again?"

I wait for a pinprick of envy to emerge, but it doesn't come.

Martin finishes up his lunch and walks over to me.

"You ready for the next one?"

"I don't think I am," I sigh. "Between yesterday in the pool and the jellyfish today, I don't think scuba diving is for me."

"I don't believe that. You just got a lit'le unlucky on your first go around, that's all. I'll make you a deal. The best deal in Thailand. You go out there for a second dive, and I'll be your buddy for the rest of your certification. I'm comin' up on my 1,000th dive. We'll hit it during your certification. It would be an honor to dive my 1,000th dive with you."

I look at my stings and bite my lip, my resignation trumped by Martin's nonjudgmental kindness.

"Only if you promise that you won't swim too far away from me."

"I promise."

I finish my soul-hugging bowl of curry, and our little diving crew heads back into the sea. I stay close to Martin, bumping into him while I look out for more jellies. My inhales and exhales startle me as the sound of air flowing through the regulator echoes in my ears, providing me with direct feedback about my heightened mental state. The only sound I hear is my anxious breathing, and its irregular rhythm distracts me. I can't pay attention to Martin or the skills I am supposed to be learning when I am busy wondering how many more shallow bursts of breath I have before I use up all of my oxygen and suffocate in the Indian Ocean.

So I count. Three seconds in. Five seconds out. I hold my arms across my chest and kick as I chant to myself.

One, two, three.

One, two, three, four, five.

One, two, three.

One, two, three, four, five.

Next to Martin, I settle into a rhythm, listening to my breath as we kick toward the rock. Sea anemones sway in the current, reminding me of the way the rice paddies rippled in the Sekinchan wind. Schools of fish that look like dinner plates flutter around us and skinny barracudas dart off in the distance. I keep my eye on the rock. As long as Martin and the rock are both within my line of sight, maybe I am safe.

I kick on, holding my arms close to my body lest there are any rogue jellies still floating around. Seawater trickles into my mask, and I don't dare tip my head back to clear it. I am not ready to see what lurks in the open ocean, so I let the salty droplets soften the edges of my vision, slowly narrowing my underwater world, one whimpering kick at a time.

19

Ross calls me over as I am walking past his bungalow, my right ankle swollen and hot from a jellyfish sting.

"You okay?" he asks, crossing one long leg over the other while lighting a cigarette.

"You're too smart for that," I say, referring to his cigarette.

"I have a rule. I only smoke in Asia. Because it's part of life here. It's too hot to do anything else so you sit around, shoot the shit, drink stale beer, and smoke. It's fantastic. When we go to Europe," Ross takes a satisfying drag, exhales, "I'll stop."

I raise an eyebrow.

"You want to sit?" Ross grabs a chair from inside his bungalow and drags it out onto his porch. We angle the chairs toward the ocean sloshing a few hundred feet away.

"What's up with you?" Ross asks. "I don't see you around that much."

"I don't want to be around that much, I guess. I find the group dynamic to be . . . "

"An overwhelming shitshow?"

"Batshit. Or maybe *baht* shit, since we're in Thailand."

"So that's why you disappeared in Malaysia."

"Partly."

Ross takes a drag, bounces his long foot. He moves with a sort of fluid grace that seems to slow down time. If any part of his Remote Year experience is destabilizing, he doesn't show it. Instead he commands a steady, almost ethereal attention, settling my turbulence like a good chunk of ginger settles seasickness.

"Can I tell you something?" I ask him. "I know we don't know each other well, but I feel like you might actually kind of get it given your work at the suicide hotline."

Ross straightens up in his chair and nods. "Go ahead."

"I spent almost fifteen years on antidepressants and only got off them when I found out about Remote Year. And I'm not handling the transition all that well." By the time the last word is out of my mouth, tears are running down my face.

"Shit," Ross says. "I don't know what to say, but I can see where you thought I was your best option."

I chuckle and wipe the tears.

"It's been months since I got off the last drug and the intensity of everything is still jacked up to 100. It's like turning up all the filters in Photoshop until the photo no longer resembles reality. I'm fine one minute and sobbing the next. Everything hurts. Everything is overwhelming. Everything is loud. So loud. Did you notice how loud Kuala Lumpur was?"

"Not particularly. Didn't you live in New York?"

"The drugs were like earmuffs. As soon as they were gone, New York was a nightmare."

"And that's why you fucked off to a rice paddy in the middle of nowhere, Malaysia. I was wondering why, of all places, that's where you chose to go."

"Now you know."

"Now I know."

"Don't tell anyone."

"I won't."

We sit in silence for a few minutes and watch the ocean sparkle in the sunlight. I am relieved to have told someone.

Ross breaks the silence. "Well, you inspired me. I'm going to pull a Brooke and fuck off somewhere without telling anyone. Maybe one of the other Thai islands. Maybe up north somewhere."

"For how long?"

"Five or six days, maybe a week."

"You going to tell anyone where you're going?"

"Nope."

"You should probably tell someone."

"You didn't."

"Fair point."

Ross points to my swelling ankle.

"That's looking like it might be infected. You should probably go get a Z-pack of antibiotics at the pharmacy. This is Thailand; you don't need a prescription."

"You think?"

"Oh yeah."

"It was getting a little better and then I took a walk on the beach and it started killing me."

Ross lifts his pant leg. His right ankle is fat and wrapped in gauze.

"Oh no, not you too," I say. "Motorbike?"

"Lost control as I was slowing down and used my foot as a kickstand. I think a bunch of sand got in it, and now it's all purple and swollen. The Z-packs cost like ten bucks."

"Fine. I'll go get myself a Z-pack. Only because it hurts to walk and I'm going a little stir crazy in the bungalow."

"Rent a motorbike like everyone else."

"You mean crash like everyone else?"

"Fair point."

Ross puts out his cigarette and smooths back his black hair. "Tell you what, I'll leave my keys to the moto with you when I leave. I rented the thing for the month. Use it if you want, or just make sure it doesn't get stolen."

"Deal."

Ross and I get up and hobble to his bungalow. He grabs his motorbike keys from inside and tosses them to me.

"Have fun on the rice paddy, or wherever it is that you end up," I say.

"I will. See you when I get back. Don't crash."

"Very funny," I say, limping away.

~~~~~~~~~~

A bottle of DEET explodes in my bag and marinates my cell phone in diethyltoluamide. I need to get to an electronics repair shop six miles away in Thongsala, the hub of Koh Phangan. I have only two options: hail a taxi or get on a motorbike. A taxi will cost me around 200 baht, the cell phone somewhere in the thousands. I hobble to an ATM and try to withdraw the cash, but the ATM errors out. It's empty. I go to another ATM right next door and try that one. It is also empty. My ankle throbs as I shuffle down the main road, past half a dozen stray dogs sleeping in the middle of the street, over puddles from last night's rainstorm, past a stand of smelly durian fruit, and into the local 7-Eleven. The store has air conditioning and walking into it is like plunging into an ice bath after an hour in a sauna. I go to the back and try the ATM, but the damn thing is tapped out too. There is an actual bank in Thongsala, but I am short the 200 baht I need to get there by taxi. On this cash-only island, it seems Remote Year has bled the ATMs dry.

I go back to my bungalow and find the keys to Ross's motorbike. Matilda takes a leap off the bed and flies onto my shorts with wide, outstretched claws. She latches on and dangles from my thighs, pathetic meows signaling that she's hungry. And hangry, apparently.

I let her dangle off my shorts as I open a can of tuna. She loses it when the smell of fish fills the bungalow and digs her back claws into my thigh, trying to break free. But her little claws are stuck in my shorts and the more she struggles, the harder she digs in. I pry her off my shorts one claw at a time. When I finally get her free she scrambles to the counter and sticks her entire face in the can of tuna while blood drips down my leg.

"Thanks, Matilda," I tell her, dabbing my bleeding thigh with a paper towel. "Don't forget to tip your waitress."

Matilda ignores me and I leave her whisker-deep in tuna while I put a few Band-Aids over my pierced skin. I pocket the motorbike keys and go next door, where another neighbor, Duncan, is working away on his front porch with a frosty Chang beer and a view of the sea. Duncan is a six-foot-four WordPress developer with a mess of sandy-brown hair and the personality of an excited lamb. He gets along with everyone and spends his free time helping others set up websites for their side projects and travel blogs. He also rides motorcycles, real motorcycles, and so far, he's one of the only Remotes who hasn't crashed a motorbike.

"What happened to your leg?" Duncan asks, looking away from his laptop and at my bandaged thigh.

"Cat," I say, without elaborating.

I climb the stairs to Duncan's porch, each step throbbing between my swollen ankle and bloody leg.

"Duncan, I need a favor. You're the only one I trust to help me with this."

"Need a website?" he says with a wink.

"No, not that. I want to learn how to drive a motorbike. Could you teach me?"

"Sure! They're really easy."

"But everyone seems to be bad at it."

"They're moving too fast around the corners. The motorbike's tires can't handle dirt roads and tight turns. That's why I rented a dirt bike. I'll show you."

Duncan closes his computer and we go to the parking lot, where his dirt bike and Ross's motorbike are parked. He compares the hefty, textured tires on his bike to the bald, flimsy tires on the motorbike, then straddles the seat and gets to the lesson.

"This is easy, Brooke. I promise. You've got the front brake on the left and the rear brake on the right. Ignition. Kickstand. And the gas on the right handle." Duncan turns on the bike and revs the engine by rotating the right handle. The sound rushes through my body and I start breathing faster.

Maybe I should just rent a bicycle.

"So here's the most important part," Duncan says. "When you're getting ready to go, make sure you have your brake on. What keeps happening to people is they hit the gas without the brake and go shooting forward. Then they crash. So ease off the brake as you start to accelerate. Make sense?"

I nod without blinking.

"It's easier to just do it," he says, getting off the bike. "Here, get on and give it a shot."

I take a deep breath, put on a helmet, and mount the bike. The seat is hot and the vinyl fabric sticks to my skin. I am sweating from every pore, my head spinning from both nerves and the beating sun. I am not just learning to drive a motorbike. I am directly disobeying my mother. I may be thirty years old and on the other side of the world, but I swear I can feel her waking from a deep sleep, wondering why she's suddenly unsettled.

Duncan holds the bike steady while I orient myself. I turn on the ignition, kick up the kickstand, and hold the rear brake. I push the start button and the bike jumps to life.

"You're doing great!" Duncan says. "Now ease off the brake and turn the handle for a little gas."

I rotate the right handle millimeter by millimeter.

"A little more."

I rotate it a little more.

"Keep going. Ease off the brake."

The bike putts forward and I slam on the brake.

"That's it!" Duncan shouts. "Do it again!"

I go through the same motions and take the bike farther down the parking lot, stopping every few feet until I feel comfortable enough to let the bike scoot along in a circle around a grinning Duncan. When I complete the circle I come to a stop, my knuckles white despite never topping eight kilometers per hour.

"Want to take it out on the main road?" Duncan asks.

"No, I do not," I say. "But I guess I have to."

"I'll follow you on my bike and watch. Just take it out a kilometer or so. You're going to have to pick up some speed. Keep it around twenty-five kilometers per hour and turn around when you're ready."

"That's like lightning death speed."

"It's a school zone."

I putt putt out of the parking lot and through the jungle leading to the main road. Duncan follows me on his dirt bike and pulls up next to me when we hit the intersection.

"You'll need to give it enough gas on the turn, more than you were just using in the parking lot. Ready?" I gulp, hold my breath, and turn onto the main road. The bike swerves and I grip the handles and give it some gas and the bike levels out. I clench my jaw and squeeze the handles until my hands cramp, my vision narrowing while I look for stray dogs, coconuts, or potholes. I am going only fifteen kilometers per hour, but my chest tightens at the thought of picking up speed. My reservoirs of grit and courage are empty, the feeling of pure terror not escaping into the wind but settling in my throat.

Dad, I need you. Help me. Keep me safe.

I give the throttle a turn and the wind picks up, whipping the sweat off my arms. The town around me begins to pass by in a blur, each palm tree and shack and bystander blinking away as quickly as it appeared. The sound of the tiny Thai town disappears into the roar of the motorbike's engine, and the faster I go the more I seem to float off the asphalt. I grip harder, fly faster, and take the bike up to forty kilometers per hour. As I give the bike gas, I hear my father's voice as if he were patching through a headset tucked into my helmet.

"It's goddamn fun, isn't it?"

"You bastard," I whisper. "I can't believe someone else had to teach me this."

"Your mother."

"I know."

"She loves you."

"I know."

"We loved you."

"I miss you."

"I know."

I come to a stop and turn the bike around. The Southeast Asian heat envelops me and I look down the road. Duncan is in the distance, waiting for me to return. I have ridden 400 meters, maybe, but the grin across my face belongs to the part of me that just completed a bigger journey. I am so excited that I may as well have scooted across the country.

"You did it!" Duncan cheers as I come back.

"I did it!" I am still shaky, but this time with elation rather than fear. "So that's it? I'm ready to take this thing all the way to Thongsala?"

"Yep. You'll be there in no time."

I thank Duncan and wave goodbye as he revs his dirt bike and speeds into the jungle. I settle myself back on the motorbike and take off in the direction of Thongsala, smirking at the thought of telling my mother about my two-wheeled transgression. She won't be happy about it, I know. But maybe it will help when I tell her I wasn't alone, that Dad showed up and wrapped his big hands around mine. He rode with me, not just on those 400 meters, but all the way to Thongsala and back, reminding me not just to look at what's right in front of me, but to keep my eyes up, always looking ahead.

20

"Gather round, mates." Martin calls Mike and me to join him on the bow. Val and Mat got into a motorbike accident and are too scraped up to dive, so it's just Mike and me on the boat along with a few dive masters-in-training. We are about to make our second dive of the day after spending the last two hours on the surface, watching the sky turn dark while an angry ocean tossed the boat like a rubber ducky in a sloshing bath. Mike makes his way to the bow, but turns gray and stops to dry heave into the sea. I can't watch him so I curl myself into a ball and stare at Sail Rock, at the unmoving horizon, and push away the thought of throwing up into my regulator fifty feet below the surface of the ocean.

"Martin, I don't know if I should be doing this," Mike says, head hanging off the side of the boat. The sky opens up and rain starts to fall. Other boats start to pull up their anchors, pack up their buoys, and leave Sail Rock.

"I promise the lot of you," Martin says, "as soon as you hit the water the seasickness will melt away. Underneath the surface, it's calm. Some of the best divin' happens during shit weather. Now let's go over the skills we need to practice so we can get in the water and get the fook out of the rain."

Martin walks us through underwater navigation, using the compass attached to our BCDs.

"I need to know you can orient yourselves in shit visibility so you don't get lost in the ocean. You think you know where you are, but you don't. So we'll all go down together and kick around to the other side of Sail Rock. Then I'm gonna need each of you to kick in a square. You'll take twen'ty kicks, look at the compass, turn ninety degrees, kick another twen'ty kicks, and so on. While each of you is kicking in a square, the other will have to control their buoyancy and stay in one place. Got it?"

We nod.

"But if we see a whale shark, forget everything I just said and follow me!"

"Have you seen any whale sharks around here?" Mike asks, the color returning to his face.

"Oh yeah, mate. We get a few e'vry year. They're not actually sharks. Just a big fookin' fish. Biggest fish in the sea. Gentle giants, they are. Don't want anything more to do with humans other than to play for a lit'le bit."

I zip up my wetsuit and plop down on a bench to hook myself into my BCD.

"Martin," I ask, "isn't your 1,000th dive coming up?"

Martin tugs at the strap on his oxygen tank and waits a beat before responding. A soft smile emerges on his face. He bobs his head in gratitude and places his right hand over his heart.

"Yes, yes it is, mates. This is my 1,000th dive."

"We have to celebrate!" Mike cheers.

"Tradition says I'm supposed to take my 1,000th dive in nothin' but me birthday suit. But seein' as you're still gettin' certified, I'll save that for another dive."

Martin waddles over to me, his fins smacking the wet boat deck with each floppy step. He looks me up and down, goes through each BWARF step of the buddy check and puts his hands on my shoulders.

"You ready, mate?"

"You sure we're okay in this weather?" I ask.

"Yep, I'm sure. You won't even notice what's happening up here when you get down there."

"I don't know why I can't get used to this." I tighten my BCD as tight as it will go.

"I'll be right with you the whole time. Just keep those breaths slow. You're doing great. Now take my hand and let me help you on up."

Martin pulls me to a standing position and steadies me as I stagger top heavy to the edge of the boat. I stride off the deck and fall to the ocean, where Mike is already waiting. Martin and the other dive masters follow us in.

We descend.

I cross my arms over my chest and stay to Martin's right, keeping him in my peripheral vision. Sail Rock emerges out of the blue and with it a flurry of movement. Visibility is about ten meters, enough to keep Sail Rock in easy sight. I steady my breath, counting one, two, three, one, two, three, four, five, one, two, three, one, two, three, four, five. Martin was right about the weather on the surface not affecting the waters below. A storm may be brewing above us, but down here it is calm, almost orderly. The fish go about their day-to-day business, darting in and out of coral while the sea anemones sway. Still, I am on high alert, constantly checking my air supply, looking around for jellyfish, and keeping Martin within sight.

We pick up speed and kick around the corner. I stay close to Sail Rock and look at it as we turn, but when I straighten out on the other side of the rock, I turn to Martin and he is gone. My heart rate shoots up and I forget about counting and I breathe faster, faster. I spin around and think I make a 180-degree turn, but Sail Rock isn't on my left and isn't on my right. There is only dark and open ocean and I look up—nothing. I look down—nothing. I turn around to find Sail Rock and as I make the turn I see a figure in the distance and I swim toward it. It is Martin with Mike pulling at his fin. Mike is pointing out into the ocean, out into the darkness. Martin looks into the deep. I kick over and follow their gaze. A massive creature is suspended in the water, not ten meters away.

A whale shark.

Martin kicks like hell toward the spotted creature and I follow, the adrenaline pushing my anxious breath out of my mind. The whale shark seems to know we are coming and kindly slows its pace to let us catch up.

We let Sail Rock fall out of sight as we swim alongside the whale shark, circling around one another with curiosity and awe. His body appears to be painted like a ceramic bowl, its creamy, smooth, white belly contrasted against its gray back, dotted with white spots scattered like stars in the night sky. Dozens of remoras cling to its skin, giving the whale shark a full body scrub while gaining protection from predators.

Fear drops out of me and dissolves into the expanse. My mind goes blank—all that exists above the surface and all I am on land falling away, my world focused on nothing but this thirty-foot, 20,000-pound creature. There is nothing left in me but awe, no moment that matters more than this. My body becomes one with the water, my lungs drawing in oxygen from my tank as if it is a part of me.

I reach out for the whale shark, knowing not to touch him but wanting to get as close to him as I can. I take a slow lap around him and watch as his golf-ball-sized eyes, charmingly small compared to the rest of its massive body, follow me as I swim toward its face. I kick in front of him and dive down about ten feet before flipping on my back. I turn over just in time to see the whale shark float slowly above me. I lose all conscious connection to my body and my breath and fall into the rhythm of the whale shark, kicking at just the right speed to let him guide me to wherever he is going.

This is peace.

As its white belly swells like the underside of a canoe and takes in a wide mouthful of plankton-rich seawater, I start to cry. But for the first time since getting off all the drugs, these are tears of joy. I am overcome with awe in this moment, a moment of beauty and serenity serving as an equal and opposite force against the worst moments of this past year. What began thirty floors above a Manhattan sidewalk ultimately led me here, twenty meters underneath the surface of the sea. With each episode of rage, pain, and depression, there was always part of me that knew I could bear it because as long as I was still breathing, I had to bear it. As long as I didn't go out of my window, I was forced to push through day after day. I always wondered why I bore this pain when there didn't seem to be anything in the world beautiful enough to fight the sorrow.

But here in the presence of this magnificent creature somewhere in the Gulf of Thailand, detached from all of my senses except the sound of my breath, I find a moment of wonder that can battle the hopelessness, and win. It is temporary, I know, but it exists. Maybe, just maybe, all of the bad days behind me do not have to add up to a bad life.

My pool of salty tears begins to cloud my vision. I keep kicking, and without thinking about it I tip my head back, press my mask to my forehead, and exhale out of my nose, clearing my mask of the tears. I watch as the bubbles float away from me and break against the whale shark's skin. Like all the painful moments before this, I know there are moments to come that will not be this easy. This one, right now, is easy. I have one. I have this one.

And one can always become two.

I sign up for my advanced scuba certification as soon as we return to the dive shop. The whale shark gifted me peace, and now I want it again and again. I dive as much as I can afford to throughout my remaining days in Thailand, accepting the gift the ocean delivers. Each ball of baitfish, each eel snaking its way through the reef, and each shrimp opens me up to a sense of wonder. As I begin to recognize the feeling of beauty and curiosity under the water, it's like I can hear the island surroundings speak to me too. The smooth, white sands, brilliant sunsets, and splash of ocean waves all begin to fight against the withdrawal that still lingers. Instead of seconds of peace, I get minutes. Precious minutes.

But as soon as old water bottles wash up on the beach and the clangs and bangs of construction cut through the quiet and drill into my ears, I am pulled back into dark reality with a force holding a magnifying glass against my mind, singeing me into the sand until I am burned into an unrecognizable mass. Each time I am back in this wounded place, still surrounded by paradise, I am reminded that I am not healed. Anxiety rushes back in and I worry about going to Cambodia and leaving the safety of Martin and the dive shop.

I already know Phnom Penh, the capital city where we're staying, is nothing but noise. Word got around about my inability to handle the chaos of Kuala Lumpur, and people keep warning me that Phnom Penh will be worse because of what happened there. From 1975 to 1979, the Khmer Rouge regime killed two million of its own people, effectively exterminating an entire culture and demolishing the country's infrastructure. Now it's a reckless place, caught between the destruction of the past and the relentless march forward into the future. Even Ross, who has spent significant time in Cambodia, wonders whether it's a good idea for me to go.

I decide to give the country a shot only when I find out a couple I know from my gym in New York City, Javi and Justine, will happen to be traveling through Phnom Penh right when I am slated to show up. Instead of going on a traditional honeymoon after their wedding, Javi and Justine took a year-long sabbatical from their NYC lives and turned a honeymoon into a worldwide honey-year. While I am still in the early stages of my trip, they are on the last leg of theirs. We will overlap for only two days, so if I decide the city is too much for me, I can follow in their footsteps and get out. Where I'd go, I don't know, but knowing I have an exit plan makes the transition easier to bear.

The day before Remote Year is scheduled to fly to Cambodia, I go to the dive shop to say goodbye to Martin. He sits on top of one of the wooden picnic tables, smoking as usual, with one leg curled underneath him while the other dangles off the edge. His eyes are heavy, whether from booze or lack of sleep or sadness, I can't quite tell. My heart aches when I see him sitting there alone. Over the course of the month, this forty-five-year-old, categorically homeless man with a diving addiction has become my de facto best friend. Though I never knew why Martin was drawn to me more so than the others, I know there is something about our relationship that hits him hard in the heart.

I don't want to leave him.

"Is it about that time?" he asks, a cloud of smoke swirling around him.

I nod and think of the first time I saw Martin, just as he was stepping off the ferry that brought us both to Koh Phangan. He was coming home after years away. I was wondering if I would ever find a home within myself. Neither one of us had any clue we'd become entangled in each other's return.

Martin reaches behind him, grabs a plastic container, and holds it out to me. I turn the container over in my hands and release the seal. Inside is a brand-new dive mask.

"I had it specially ordered for you," Martin says, his eyes a little misty. "I get a lot of people comin' through 'ere, you know. I'm really gonna miss you. You and me, we're family now. So whenever you use that dive mask, think of me. And I sure hope you get to use it."

At a loss for words, I give Martin a long hug.

"You can always come back home," he says.

I nod and squeeze him tight, hoping one day I'll know he's right.

21

Our plane lands in Phnom Penh at sunset. As soon as the doors open, my mouth goes dry and all I taste is dust. It is a stark contrast to the wet, salty Thai air that seemed to hydrate me from the inside out. Here, mere minutes after landing in Cambodia, every cell in my body shrivels and begs for water.

I open my bag, looking for a bottle of something to quench the thirst. Perched on top of my toiletries is the dive mask Martin gave me as we said goodbye last night. Just hours out of Thailand my heart already aches for the quiet of the cerulean water. I still can't shake the feeling that something about Cambodia isn't safe for me, like I'm too fragile to function in a place with so much pain. I have just begun to find moments of life that can battle against the darkness. I'm worried I haven't had enough practice living in the light and I'll step off the plane, tap right into the grief of this place, and fall back into the horror and pain and sorrow of every perished soul that came before me. What if, this time, I can't shake *them* off?

As I pay for my visa and walk onto Cambodian soil, I feel like I'm entering into the Colosseum. All I've been through, all the work I've done, is put on display for the souls of the departed that fill the seats. They watch me as I step out of the airport, and the chaos of the city nearly knocks me flat. They see my chest tighten as tuk-tuks and motorbikes swerve all around me, stoplights and traffic signs mere suggestion rather than doctrine. They know I weaken when I arrive at my Remote Year apartment and look out the window to find a construction crew within spitting range. With each screech of metal on metal, they wonder if I will crumble.

I shove earplugs into my ears, put on my headphones, and pipe my trusty brown noise through the speakers. I get into bed without bothering to unpack, waiting for sleep to come.

~~~~~~~~~~~

I wake up the next morning with a familiar sense of doom. My mouth is dry as sandpaper and every cell in my body is screaming *get out, get out.* But instead of fighting it, instead of being scared, I strap on a mental seat belt and prepare for it. I've been on this ride before, and if nothing else, I'm learning that what goes down eventually comes up. Who knows how long this bout of waves will last, but at least I know I will survive it.

My Phnom Penh apartment is dark, with a single window looking toward a wall so close I can reach my hand out and touch it. None of the appliances work quite right. The refrigerator opens into the couch. A television is pushed into the only available corner, but there isn't an outlet anywhere nearby to plug it in. There is a large, heavy jug of potable water on the counter, but no pump to get the water out. When I try to gently tip a stream of water into a cup, the jug topples over and spills all over the kitchen floor. I use a scratchy, frayed towel to sop up the mess and make a mental note to ask Javi and Justine if they know of anywhere else in this part of the world where I could ride out November.

I toss the soaked towel into the stained bathtub and gather my gym bag. The plan is to meet Javi and Justine at a gym that caters to expats, a mile or so south of my apartment. I step out of the apartment building and hail a tuk-tuk. In any other part of the world, I would have walked. But here walking is impossible. Sidewalks are nonexistent and, if they do exist, they are in dangerous disrepair. One step on a loose piece of concrete could plunge you into a pile of broken glass, mangling a foot into looking like something out of a meat grinder.

My tuk-tuk bumps down unkempt roads and I hold my bag to my chest, clutching it a little tighter each time we come to a stop. Remote Year warned us to keep our bags close and to put our phones away while riding in a tuk-tuk. Phnom Penh is notorious for snatch-and-grab robberies. The moving tuk-tuk gives a false sense of security, but when a passenger is fiddling with their iPhone, someone scoots by the tuk-tuk on a moto and grabs the shiny phone right out of the rider's hands.

Tuk-tuk robbery isn't the most elegant of crimes, but it does keep me on high alert, forcing me into the present. I notice how my throat burns as my lungs fill with dust kicked up by tuk-tuks in the dry season, and how my vision narrows at the sound of construction rattling all around me. When the driver stops at a corner in the general vicinity of the gym, I feel each pore open up. I am sticky yet parched. Wide awake but exhausted to the bone. Forced into the moment yet aching to numb it all.

Next door to the gym, a man cuts tile with an electric handsaw. Across the way, a few men make tedious progress as they attempt to demolish an entire building foundation with nothing but a sledgehammer. Around the corner, I watch a man chip paint with a screwdriver. My heart beats faster, each breath shallower than the one before. I hope for relief when I walk into the gym, but the bubble tarp serving as the roof provides no protection from the beating sun or the cacophony of construction.

I feel a mounting pressure in my head as I look around, somewhat comforted by the rusted equipment and '90s hip-hop that remind me of my gym back in New York. A small man, clearly American, steps away from a barbell and introduces himself. His name is Ben, and he'll be coaching our class. A power tool roars outside and the pressure in my head sharpens. Water. I need water.

"Where around here can I get a coconut?" I ask Ben.

"Oh, there are guys walking around with carts full of coconuts around here. If you head toward the Russian Market . . . do you know where the Russian Market is?"

I shake my head. "I got in yesterday. I don't know where anything is."

"If you leave the gym and head left, go down a few blocks and make a right, then another left. Go a few blocks more and you'll see a big market. There should be some guys selling coconuts there. It shouldn't cost you over 1,000 riel. If it does, they're trying to rip you off."

I thank him, walk out of the gym, and immediately forget where I was supposed to go. I am also wearing workout shorts that reveal meaty thighs the size of most Cambodians' waists, so I'm not interested in wandering into a busy market filled with leering eyes. But I need the electrolyte-filled liquid gold inside of a coconut, and I need it now.

I turn down the first street I come across and, like magic, a young man in a checkered button-down shirt scoots toward me on a motorized bike, carting a bed full of coconuts. I flag him down and he pulls over, unruffled by the white girl in short-shorts. I hold up one finger. He opens a Styrofoam cooler housing ice-cold coconuts, pulls a machete from the depths of his cart, and in three swift thwacks pops off the top of the coconut. The man pushes a straw through its flesh and hands me my purchase. I give him a 1,000-riel bill, wave goodbye, and trot back to the gym cradling my coconut under one arm.

"You found a coconut," Ben says as I walk back in, the ends of his mustache dancing as he smiles.

"I did." The coconut is sour and fermented, far less palatable than the sugar-sweet coconuts in Thailand. Still, I suck the liquid down.

I hear a clunk behind me and turn to see Javi and Justine. I forget all about my sour coconut and, for the first time since leaving Koh Phangan, my spirits lift.

Javi gives me a big hug and, after exchanging a few pleasantries, gets right to the point.

"We've only got twenty-four hours here. So after we work out, we're going to grab lunch and then go straight to the Killing Fields. You should come!"

The moment of ease scampers away as quickly as it came when I remember I am in a country synonymous with recent, brutal genocide. I know I can't be here, in Phnom Penh, without visiting the final resting place for tens of thousands of Cambodians who were killed by Pol Pot and his murderous regime. I know this is bigger than me, that my mind and my withdrawal and my problems have to be set aside for a few hours in order to pay homage to those who perished. I also know I am scared of what I might find there and of what might be stirred up within me. Thailand showed me I'm teetering on the precipice between breakthrough and breakdown. Is it reckless to present myself to more pain, to *them*?

You are already here, in this energy. Feel it. Face it. Follow where it leads.

I decide to get it all over with and join Javi and Justine at the Killing Fields. The hour-long ride will give us time to catch up, and it will help to do this with friends. Maybe if I face them by choice, I can separate myself from them. Maybe *they* can exist alongside me in harmony, rather than dissonance. Maybe we can both break through and finally be at rest.

~~~~~~~~~~~~~~

The wind stands still on the banks of the Killing Fields. Dust hangs in the muggy air as the tuk-tuk driver comes to a halt in a precious patch of shade.

Far away from the center of Phnom Penh, birdsongs chime through the rolling hills. Somewhere in the distance, the sound of children's laughter echoes in my ears. Still, the silence here is heavy, turning my stomach with each passing second. Javi exchanges phone numbers with the driver. The driver doesn't speak English and Javi doesn't speak Khmer, but somehow they decide on a time for us all to gather together again. The tuk-tuk turns in a wide circle and leaves us in a cloud of dust.

If you didn't know what happened here, this place might be described as beautiful. At first look, it is an oasis of green in the middle of endless miles of dirt. A Buddhist stupa stands just behind the entrance, its ornate, gold-and-silver roof glistening in the clear sky. Tall trees with thick trunks tower over the grounds, providing shade for winding walking bridges where stray puppies take refuge in the cover. But around 20,000 souls perished on these particular grounds, and killing fields just like this one are scattered throughout the country. Not all are marked by gates. Most are simply pockmarked stretches of land, the rolling hills built of bones, not soil.

Outside this entrance, outside the bloodshed, a few stands sell drinks and snacks. It is odd to see vendors parked outside of a place where unimaginable atrocities occurred. I think of the juicy oranges sold just outside the ruins of Pompeii, so close to the stone walls that a good arm and a little aim could heave one right over the barrier and into 1,900-year-old ashes. I remember visiting Auschwitz after graduating college. On one side of the Polish gates, a stand sold bottled water and ice cream—on the other side, manicured grass and a fresh coat of paint on the gas chambers. Through I logically understood the grounds needed to be landscaped, the buildings renovated, and structures replicated in order to preserve history as memory fades and survivors leave this Earth, I could never quite square the emotional circle of intentionally maintaining a monument to profound evil. And I certainly didn't understand why anyone would want to eat something as playful as ice cream at a concentration camp.

Now I stand on the other side of the world, outside the gates of yet another one of humanity's worst eras, staring at more icy coconuts. Liquid luxury mere feet away from a tower of human bones. I go to the gate, wrap my hands around the metal, and put my forehead to the bars. I am dehydrated from the unrelenting Cambodian heat. But to drink a coconut in front of *them*, to nourish myself with light in the presence of dark? How can we both coexist?

I forget the coconut, walk inside the gates, and part from Javi and Justine. Now that I'm here, I know I need to do this alone. I put on my headset and walk through the grounds, listening as my audio guide clicks from one grisly piece of history to another. When Pol Pot rose to power in 1975, he aimed to turn Cambodia into a cashless, agrarian utopia. He promised peace after years of living in the shadow of the Vietnam War, but that promise was never fulfilled. Cambodians were rounded up en masse and sent to the countryside to perform forced agricultural labor, their possessions seized, their money confiscated.

They were packed into trucks and transported to the once-sleepy village of Choeung Ek, now known as the Killing Fields, where they were slaughtered and dumped into shallow, crowded graves. I am careful as I walk across this hallowed land. The dirt paths are scattered with teeth, hidden in plain sight among the pebbles. Swatches of bloody clothing, deflated in the absence of a long-decomposed body, peek out of the dirt like exposed roots. Deep inside the grounds, there is a tree where babies were held by their ankles and—in front of their mothers—swung headfirst into a blood-soaked trunk.

And still, the hills are green and rich and the sky is clear-blue. There is a lake tucked deep into the land, covered in flourishing lily pads. I find a bench on the water's edge and sit, taking off my audio guide to listen to the birds singing in the trees. Fat chickens roam free, pecking at scraps, while lizards bathe in slivers of sun. A frog croaks and hops from lily pad to lily pad. Free of the intruding amphibian, each leaf shivers, then settles.

It shouldn't be this beautiful here.

I start to heave, then sob, not only because I am surrounded by death, but because I am surrounded by life, too. It is all here, all at once, existing in bittersweet balance. All this time I saw the two as separate entities within me, one unable to thrive in the presence of the other. So I spent half my life choosing to imitate death, to get myself as close to it as I could in order to numb the sting of living. Death was the easier choice. Envy the prey, not the vulture.

But life and death are opposite doors into the same room. As I feel into these perished souls, these beautiful souls, I wonder whether I would have felt this place if I was still on all the drugs. I didn't shed a tear at Auschwitz. The whole experience washed off me like a drab history lesson, the black-and-white headshots of gaunt prisoners no more meaningful to me than the faces in someone else's yearbook. My soul was separate then. Not so much protected by the drugs but suspended in a state of permanent shelter, the doors to both darkness and light slammed shut.

Only the window ever offered a way out.

The tears fall and I feel a familiar pull, down into the scratchy, wooden bench. My limbs go heavy and my edges wane.

I close my eyes and think of Alan's instructions, pouring compassion into every crackling part of me, and into every shattered part of *them*. I let the buzz pulse throughout my body, let the edges fall all the way away, let the phrases come to me in a steady stream of consciousness.

"I'm so sorry you're scared," I whisper. I keep my eyes closed and wait. From somewhere deep within me: *"I'm so sorry you're scared."*

"I'm so sorry we couldn't transform your pain."

"We are all born into our own story."

"I'm so sorry you are trapped in this place."

"We stay gated so you remember."

"I'm so sorry you didn't know you could leave at any time."

"We need to be shown how."

"I'm so sorry you didn't know how to begin."

"You have already begun."

A rooster squawks and my eyes flutter open. The heat persists, but a chill runs down my spine. Tears of sorrow and gratitude erupt from my soul and I know I am here, fully in my body. I am, *they* are, alive. No matter the fate, this land, this country, these people, they persist. And though my own war is small and internal, the enemy none other than myself, I too can only march forward.

I stand and walk back to the entrance. I return my audio guide and turn toward the stupa, rising tall over the hills. What you can't see from the outside is that the stupa is lined with skulls, arranged one on top of another based on the kind of fatal blow each victim received. One wall built of gunshots. Another made of blunt objects to the head. Each skull so small, yet it once held a whole world.

I turn back to the gate and see Javi and Justine are waiting with the tuk-tuk driver. As I step through the gate, I know something is different. There is an understanding now, that though *they* will always exist, I do not have to carry them with me.

My tongue is thick and sticky, a layer of grime begging to be rinsed off. I go to the vendor and buy a coconut and sip the bittersweet, nourishing liquid. It runs through my body and swells my parched cells, filling them with sugar and electrolytes needed to fight the heat of this place. I savor it. I feel the roughness of the coconut's shell in my palms. I dig for pulp with my straw and lick the fatty flesh from my fingers. When I am done, I wipe my hands and say "thank you" to no one in particular but to everyone—all of *them*—all at once. They will be there for me, always, if I choose to listen. And if I listen, I'm sure, I will hear them roar.

~~~~~~~~~

After I say goodbye to Javi and Justine later that day, I decide to stay in Cambodia. I owe it to myself, and to *them*, to let this place help me stitch old wounds I've been reluctant to heal. For fifteen depressed years, I built an identity on a foundation of brokenness, believing I would never have the power, strength, or will to overcome my own mind without antidepressants. Nine months of withdrawal shattered that assumption. It's been long enough now that I'm beginning to worry I am using withdrawal as a crutch to entrench myself in a new, yet still wounded, identity. The target, for a decade and a half, was depression. I thought withdrawal would dissolve the target entirely and I would emerge from this year whole and enlightened. Instead, I can feel the target moving, the warped identity of a woman in withdrawal threatening to take over.

There's no denying I am not done, that the waves of withdrawal will continue to ebb and flow. For how long, I don't know. But I can feel the conscious choice now. I can choose to create an identity around my withdrawal, viewing myself as fragile, unpredictable, and unable to handle the chaos of the world. Or I can refuse to accept that fate and instead practice radical acceptance. I can choose to trust each wave of withdrawal will pass and, in the windows in between each wave, I will have the strength to let myself bathe in the light instead of preparing for the dark. I can choose to trust that, with time, the windows will stay open longer and longer. I can choose to trust that in those times of peace, I will know where to take my next step.

So when Ross invites me to a traditional Cambodian wedding taking place in a little village about five hours outside of Phnom Penh, I perk up.

"Thought you might need to get away from all the construction in the city," Ross says.

I flash a wide, sarcastic smile and bat my eyelashes.

"You noticed I wasn't coping so well here?" I say.

"Your poker face is terrible," he says.

I drop the smile and hang my head. Though I am determined not to surrender my power to withdrawal, the symptoms still persist.

"How do you know these people?" I ask.

"My cousin lived with them for a few years while she set up a school in their village. She'll come too, so we'll have a translator."

"Whose wedding are we going to?"

"No idea," Ross says. "I'm not sure my cousin does either. It's one of those things where the whole village just shows up. We're going to have to teach you how to drink, though."

"I know how to drink." I down the rest of a lukewarm Angkor beer. "See?"

"Oh, that's cute. But no. They take shots of rice wine. *Bootleg* rice wine. It will fuck you up."

I narrow my eyes.

"There's a trick," Ross continues. "When they pour you a shot, raise the glass with everyone else. 'Choul mouy' is the word for 'cheers' in Khmer, so everyone will say that and then take the shot. Bring the shot to your lips with everyone else. Take a sip if you want, but the trick is to dump the rest of the shot into the dirt without it being obvious. Watch."

Ross pours an inch of beer into the bottom of a cup, takes a quick but dramatic sip, then flings the rest of the liquid onto the ground in one swift motion.

"But then I'll end up with a puddle of rice wine on the floor next to me," I say.

"The floor is dirt. And the alternative is alcohol poisoning in the middle of nowhere, Cambodia," Ross says.

"Comforting."

Ross crosses one long leg over the other, lights a cigarette, and shrugs.

22

I leave a sweaty workout shirt at the gym and Ben finds me on Facebook to tell me he put my shirt in the wash. It will be in the lost and found when I return, he says, and if I'd like to experience a little bit of his Phnom Penh, he's available after 5:00 p.m.

I meet him in the wet bowels of an indoor market because I'm looking for sparkly shoes.

"Cinderella shoes?" Ben smirks as he leads me past old women hacking the heads off fish, past rows of auto-part shops and a line of slot machines, and into the clothing section of the market where cheap T-shirts, knockoff jeans, and plastic flip-flops hang from every corner.

"Apparently, I'm going to a Cambodian wedding in the countryside this weekend, and I was told to buy some sparkly shoes. I don't know. I'm just following directions."

"You've been here for, what, four days? How did you get yourself invited to a local wedding?" Ben asks.

"One of my fellow Remotes invited me. He has a cousin who lives in Cambodia and helped open a school in a province near the border of Vietnam. She's going back to the countryside for a wedding and said Ross and a friend could come with."

"I hear Cambodian weddings are one hell of a party." Ben thumbs through a rack of shoes, but seems dissatisfied with the selection. He is short, like me, with reddish hues speckled throughout his sandy-brown beard. A mustache curls at the corner of his lips, giving him the air of an old-time saloon barback. His eyes are calm, kind, and gray, and I instantly like being around him.

"What about these?" Ben says, pulling out a pair of silver slippers from the bottom of the pile. They are covered in sequins.

"They are sparkly. And I was told to get sparkly. Good work."

I buy the sparkly shoes and Ben and I walk to the extent we can in Phnom Penh.

"Careful," Ben says as he leaps over a large puddle. "Whatever that puddle is, it's probably not water you want to step in."

"That much is clear," I say, staring into the brown muck. "What is it?"

Ben smirks and points to an open canal wide enough to need bridges, with a slurry of brown sludge running through it. "Well that's Shit Creek. So . . . "

I give him a death glare, look at the puddle, and consider my limited options. The puddle runs into the street, so to skirt around it would be to wander onto a busy road where tuk-tuks and motorbikes zigzag against the flow of traffic. I clutch my bag to my chest, back up, and take a running leap over the puddle.

"Great form," Ben says. "You're a pro. By the way, if something happens while you're here and you need to go to a hospital, just to go Bangkok. Even if you're unresponsive and dying, go to Bangkok."

"Thanks for the warning. You're going to need to explain to me why you chose to settle down here."

"I'm a simple guy. I can have a simple life and there are actually a lot of cool things happening here. Hungry? I'll take you to one of my favorite spots."

We dodge traffic and puddle-hop to an Australian pub. We drink Belgian beer and eat French chicken cordon bleu on mahogany stools that pull up to a bar made from reclaimed wood. A mustachioed, English bartender washes glasses by hand behind the bar. Edison light bulbs swing above us, twinkling against rows of Scotch whiskey and Kentucky bourbon. It's like Brooklyn got blackout drunk, wandered into the wrong country, and decided not to leave because the rent was so much cheaper.

Ben tells me how he came to Phnom Penh by way of Jakarta. Before that, he was in Kazakhstan, and before that, Kuwait. He likes the grit of developing countries and the freedom of living outside the cultural constraints and societal expectations of the United States. He tells me how his parents medicated him for ADHD at eight years old, which planted a seed of resentment that ultimately grew into a lifelong fight against "the establishment." He turned vegetarian to piss off Texas, then vegan to piss off vegetarians, then exclusively consumed fruit when veganism became too trendy. Throughout his teenage years and early adulthood, he didn't drink alcohol because he figured drinking was something everyone else did to rebel, so he wasn't going to drink because "rebelling by not drinking was more hard-core than rebelling by actually drinking." When he finally did decide to have a drink, it was organic red wine. He had two glasses, went home, and evaluated his life choices. The next day he ate a steak.

Now, he has just two pairs of shoes, one pair of pants, and a few T-shirts collected from gyms around the world. He pays $200 in rent and owns one towel and a single fork. He likes good coffee and beer. He doesn't use shampoo or wear deodorant.

He turns to me a few minutes into the cordon bleu and says, "Tomorrow, I'm going to get on a bus and go somewhere. I'm meeting a few friends for the weekend, but they head back to work on Sunday. There's a town called Kep a few hours away, where you can fish crabs out of the river and they'll fry them up for you right on the spot. What if, instead of staying here, you come and meet me there?"

I excuse myself and go to the restroom because I need a moment to comprehend an invitation to spend an undefined amount of time in a foreign country with a man I've been talking to for all of forty-five minutes. I wash my hands and look into the mirror, examining the face staring back at me. I haven't worn much makeup since arriving in Southeast Asia. It melts off of me whenever I step out into the heat. But my cheeks are flush with red, my lips pink and tingly. I know what I am committing to even though it has not yet been said: a romantic escapade in the Cambodian countryside with someone I will likely never see again. There is magic here, in my body and heart, awakening after years of dormancy. I want to follow this feeling wherever it takes me, across a country and away from my past and into the arms of the man sitting on the other side of this door. Ben is not my forever future, I know. I have only three more weeks in this place. But before I arrived in this country, I couldn't shake the feeling that something was going to happen to me here. Maybe that feeling wasn't so much of worry, but of significance. Maybe I was too wrapped up in my own fear to know the difference.

I return to the bar as Ben takes the last sip of his drink. He clears his throat as I settle back into my seat.

"First, I have a wedding to go to," I tell him.

The bartender clears our glasses and asks if we want another round. Ben looks at me, and I nod.

"How about when I come back, I'll come right to you?" The bartender delivers our beers, and I hold up my glass and clink its bottom against Ben's frothy mug. "Take me on an adventure."

In the dim glow of the bar's lights, Ben's mustache curls up against his cheek as he grins. I don't ask for assurance or look for any signs of doubt. I simply decide to trust this man, this stranger, with my body and my heart. There is an ease between us, safety somewhere in this man's sparkling, gray eyes. That is all I need to know.

~~~~~~~~~~

Ross and I sit on red, plastic stools in the Cambodian countryside as our hosts, Ma and Pa, record our names and passport numbers into the village ledger. Pa then takes the information, oils up his motorbike, and scoots down the potholed dirt road to announce our arrival to the local police. The reasoning behind this is twofold: The police need to know they shouldn't be alarmed by a wide-eyed white girl and ethnically ambiguous beanpole of a Ross and, more important, the villagers need to know we are Pa's guests and are not to be fucked with. This is not an area travelers pass through. Outsiders tend not to fare well in these parts.

The sun falls behind palm trees, and darkness settles across the land. Ross sits with his back against a beam and shut his eyes, seeming to relax into the stillness of the night. I light a cigarette just to hold on to a little glow of light. I let it burn down to my knuckles, occasionally tapping its ashy tip against the edge of my stool, never taking a puff.

The pain and struggle of this country seems to rise with the moon. Pol Pot and the Khmer Rouge can be whittled away during the day through manual work and day-to-day routine, but in this village the memories of battle and death are drunk down every night. The fact that Pa and the older villagers are still alive is a minor miracle. Any Cambodian over the age of fifty was directly affected by the genocide, and many of the men are killers. While Ma fled a few miles over the border to Vietnam, unsure whether her family was alive, Pa fought for the Khmer Rouge, not because he believed in the doctrine, but because it was either fight or face certain death. Every day, he said, he went to the front lines with a hundred men. Every day, maybe five came home. He got lucky, repeatedly, if luck counts as losing your left leg while being forced to slaughter your own people.

Pa tells Ross and me this story, with the help of Ross's cousin as a translator, with a sense of calm existing only in people who have seen such horrible things that they must disassociate themselves from their story to survive. Yet throughout it all, he never lost his sense of curiosity and even sneaked illegal books into his home after coming back from a day on the battlefield. He taught himself French, fully aware that if he were caught, he would be killed. The Khmer Rouge aimed to wipe out every intellectual, artist, doctor, lawyer, Christian, Buddhist, or Muslim—anyone tainted by the West. They wanted to erase the slate and start over at Year Zero, to create a society in which people worked manual labor only for the common good, without competition.

One look at Ma and Pa's faces tells me this war is not over, that it never ended. While everyone knows when it began, on April 17, 1975, the day Pol Pot led his Communist forces into Phnom Penh and seized control of Cambodia, this war did not end when Vietnam invaded Cambodia in January 1979 and the Khmer Rouge was thrown out of power. For those who survived, the war was divided into a million little pieces, each one embedded in the souls of the surviving. Much ado is made about when a story begins, but endings are never clear. Endings never end.

Pa didn't take to the bottle like so many others. Instead he turned his home into the village school, teaching French and math and a little bit of English to the village children on a whiteboard smuggled in from who knows where. At night, he sits quietly at the single, plastic table, sipping on a beer or two while neighborhood men stop by for shots of rice wine. And because Pa has foreign visitors, the men come in droves. They laugh and toast until they stumble home, blacked-out and shouting nonsense that echoes through the trees in between the howls of wild dogs. Children appear at Ma and Pa's when the drunken fighting in their home gets bad. I sit with them and together we make our way through an English workbook.

In the morning, the village men stumble out of their homes, donning stripes along their backs and chest made from pressing a coin deep into their flesh, breaking the capillaries into purple bruises believed to cure hangovers.

Eventually they wander back over and plop down on the red, plastic stools surrounding our table, glassy-eyed from the night before. A little beer. A little ice. Rice wine poured and passed around. Ross and I look at each other and, without a word, we settle into the ceremonial cheer by raising our right arm with our left hand resting on our right bicep. We nod to each other, and to the men who came for breakfast. "Choul mouy!" we cheer together.

I bring the burning liquid to my pursed lips and throw my head back along with everyone else, then fling the glass down to the ground, dumping its contents on the dirt below.

By the evening of the wedding, word spreads that foreigners will be attending. I slip on a simple cotton dress, slather myself in bug spray, and find my sparkly shoes. I haven't seen my own reflection in days and seem to be losing the battle between drugstore deodorant and body odor. Though I am in the middle of nowhere and don't know a soul at the party we are about to attend, I am self-conscious about my presence and worried about leaving the safety of Ma and Pa's property. Upon our arrival in the village, I was told not to wander off on my own. As a man, Ross was safe. I had to be careful. Women went missing in the village all the time.

"Ready?" Ross says, buttoning up his dress shirt. He looks at me as I stuff my feet into the sparkly shoes, stretching them to their limit. "Apparently we've got to walk a kilometer or so to get to the actual wedding. Are those shoes going to be okay?"

I stand, try to wiggle my toes, and can already feel where the sequins are going to rub and create a blister.

"They're not great." I pry off the shoes, shove them into my bag, and slip on a pair of sneakers for the walk. Outside, the wedding's loudspeakers blast traditional Khmer music so loud we can hear it all the way at Ma and Pa's. My chest tightens when it occurs to me how loud the music must be at the venue, and how I won't be able to leave if it becomes too much for me.

"Remind me why I'm here, again?" I ask, lacing up the sneakers for the walk.

"Because you spent your whole life on drugs and you're forcing yourself out of your comfort zone."

"Right. And yet I'm still nervous."

"Me too," Ross says. "These people party hard. Eat a lot and try and keep your beer cup about half full."

"Why half full?"

"Because if your cup is too full, they'll make you and everyone else at the table chug it. And if it's not full enough, they'll fill it up and then you'll have to chug it."

"If I don't, it'll be rude, right?"

Ross smirks. "I told you that you needed to learn how to drink like a Cambodian."

I take a breath and we venture into the night, Ma and Pa leading the way. There are no streetlights. Only moonlight illuminates whatever lurks in the shadows, and darkness envelops us as we walk. The music grows louder with each step, guiding us toward the celebration. We round a corner, and a large, white tent appears, hundreds of people crammed underneath it. The bride and groom stand outside, greeting all the guests. They are both wearing silk, the bride's ivory dress dotted with gold flowers and the groom's white suit piped in red. They are clearly expecting our arrival and bow their heads as Ross and I come by. I smile and return the bow, bringing my hands together in thanks. The bride hands me a stick of gum and goes back into the tent.

"What's this?" I whisper to Ross as we weave through the crowd of staring villagers.

"Wedding favor," he says.

We both unwrap the gum, fold it onto our tongues, and chew. It disintegrates into a mint-tinted, crumbly paste.

"Oh my god, that's awful," Ross says, searching for somewhere to spit out the granulated mess.

"I don't understand what is happening," I say, examining the green wrapper. At first glance it appears to be a standard stick of Doublemint, but a closer look reveals the truth. "Hey, Ross. It's Extramint."

Ross spits the gum into a bush. "Extramint? What?"

I hand him the wrapper, grinning.

"Oh my god. It's knockoff gum." Ross starts to laugh and hands the wrapper back to me.

"Same, same, but different. Right?" I wipe my tongue across the wrapper, trying to get rid of the taste but also delighted by the incident. There are knockoff consumer goods all over Asia, but there is something about this counterfeit chewing gum that clarifies the present moment. I notice how alert I am to the smack of my shoes on the muddy ground, to the fear that bubbles up when I see a shadow in the darkness, to the smell of one of Ross's cigarettes.

I am alive.

I reach for Ross's arm and hook my elbow into his.

"Thank you for inviting me here," I say, loud enough so he can hear me over the bellowing music.

"No problem." He blows a plume of smoke up to the night sky. "You ready?"

"Almost. I'm missing something very important." I pull off my sneakers and swap them with the sparkly shoes from my bag. My toes are crammed against the edges, and the sequins dig into my heels. But it doesn't matter anymore. The celebration will end, the blisters will heal, and I will never have to wear the shoes again. For now, the shoes are a reminder.

I am alive.

~~~~~~~

I board a bus to meet Ben the day after I return from the countryside with Ross and briefly wonder if I am making a huge mistake. I've known this guy for just a few hours, after all. But what the hell, I figure. I am already here. Besides, if I am going to get murdered in Cambodia, it may as well be by a stranger with beautiful, gray eyes and a cute butt.

I climb into the bus and find my seat next to a monk, using my giant backpack filled with random clothes and a few toiletries to prop up my legs. One year ago, that bag would have been filled with Effexor XR and Wellbutrin and Synthroid and Tetracycline and Sucralfate. Now, all I have is anti-diarrheal tablets and ibuprofen. And so far, I haven't had to touch any of it.

We drive through the Cambodian countryside as the sky turns from blue to pink to black. Outdoor markets seem to pop out of nowhere, connecting village to village, spilling people and emaciated cows and mangoes onto the single-lane road. Traffic, in the middle of nowhere, moves at a crawl. I stare out the window and into the dark eyes of women and girls stuffed onto the back of a truck bed, heading home after a day working in a garment factory. Every morning, I learned from Ma and Pa, trucks roll through the villages and pick up workers along the way, piling people into the truck bed like chickens. Every night the workers pile back in and are carted home down this stretch of road. A truck idles next to me and I count about forty people, stuffed more or less into a space five people wide and eight deep. Some of the women wave at me. Some point. Others just stare right back.

As we make our way through the congested streets and gain speed on the open road, I look through the front window of the bus and see an endless string of these trucks coming toward us in the other lane. Down each dirt path forking away from the main road, another set of trucks kicks up dust as they make their way away from factories looming in the distance. I glance at my phone, set a timer for an hour, and count.

One. Two. Three. Forty-two. Seventy-seven. One hundred fifty-five. Three hundred and eleven. Times forty—12,440 workers passed in one hour. As I stare at the number on my phone's calculator, I swipe to my day of death countdown: 19,353 days to go. That number, once an elegy to pain, now seems so full of possibility. I am proud of myself for pulling myself away from my windowsill, pushing through withdrawal, feeling this experience in all its ebbs and flows. Then I notice my cheap, cotton shirt, bought from a fashion megastore before I left the States. I feel for the tag against my torso and examine the information: Made in Cambodia.

I shrink back down into my seat.

What a privilege it is to be in this skin, on this bus, rushing toward adventure. It is a paradox, I know, to compare one person's struggle to another. All the opportunity in the world can't guarantee a carefree life, just as poverty does not doom one to inevitable suffering. Still, the life I was born into comes with a level of responsibility I am only now beginning to understand. If I have the means to step up and take care of myself, to follow a half-baked plan around the world just because something inside me was screaming to be set free, then I damn well better do it. It is my duty to take advantage of all that is afforded to me because when I do better for myself, I have the capacity to do better for others.

I know I can't save the world. I can't bridge the inequality gap, end systematic suffering, or deliver a cure for modern life. But what a waste it would have been to remain in New York, entrenched in my own bullshit, just waiting for the courage to step all the way through my window. All of this beauty, growth, and gratitude would be lost. I don't yet know what I'm going to do with it all, but I know if, nothing else, I will see through a different lens.

Next to me, the monk hums a long and pleasant tune. He is bald, middle-aged, and dressed in bright-orange robes. If he has any possessions, they are not on his person, the area under his bare feet filled with nothing but space. I wonder where he is going and if he is happy to go there.

The monk hums all the way to the countryside, to the little town of Kampot, where Ben and I are meeting. It is late by the time we arrive, and I have no way to contact Ben. Our cell phones don't work without Wi-Fi, which is spotty and hard to find in these parts. He said when I arrived to go to the giant, golden durian just a short walk from the bus stop. He would be waiting for me there, next to the enormous monument to a fruit that tastes like sweet custard but smells like old gym socks.

I swing my backpack onto my back and step off the bus. Tuk-tuk drivers swarm around me, shrieks of "Where to?" and "Fair price!" competing for my attention. I shake my head and walk away, unsure whether I am heading in the right direction. I wonder what I will do if I can't find the golden durian or if I find it and Ben isn't there. I could find a hostel, stay the night, and head back to Phnom Penh in the morning. Or maybe I could stay in Kampot for a few days, though I have no idea what is here. It might not be pleasant, but I would figure it out. That much, I know.

I didn't need to wonder. I turn a corner and see the gigantic durian, with Ben waiting for me as promised. He kisses me on the cheek and gives me an awkward but relieved hug, and, in the light of the golden, prickly fruit, I know I am safe. Just like on the phone in New York with Alan, on the rice paddy in Malaysia with Wilson, and under the sea in Thailand with Martin. Here is another person I wasn't even looking for, who appeared like a forgotten umbrella just as it starts to rain.

"You hungry?" Ben says as he slips off my backpack and swings it around his back. "There's a great little tapas place nearby."

"One of these days I'd like to eat some Cambodian food," I say, realizing that most of my diet in Cambodia has consisted of the rest of the world's cuisines.

"Then we'll go to Kep and get you those river crabs."

"Sounds perfect," I say.

He throws his arm around my shoulder and we walk into town, the glow of the golden durian lighting the way.

23

The story doesn't end here. It doesn't end in Kep, when Ben and I weave our motorbike along jet-black highways snaking through the Cambodian countryside. The anxiety I once felt riding on the back of a motorbike is gone and I relax as Ben zigzags through bright-white lane markers, leaning left and right in sync with the bike and his body. I tuck my hands underneath his shirt and let them graze over his skin as he drives us through the wilderness, the rush of wind blowing the sweat from my limbs.

It is only when my skin begins to tickle with sticky heat that I open my eyes and notice Ben slowing down. He comes to a stop in the middle of the road, and I look ahead to see an elephant walking toward us, its trunk swinging inches from the pavement. As the sweat pools down our backs, we watch in silence as the nearly ten-foot-tall creature passes us, one slow step at a time.

The story doesn't end when, on my 100th day of travel, I leave Cambodia for good. I soak Ben's shoulder in tears while a tuk-tuk driver waits for us to pull apart. In the moment, it all seems possible for us to stay together, to continue whatever this is. But the thread that bound us wears thin as the borders in between us grow and soon Ben fades from memory.

The story doesn't end in Croatia, when one day I awake into a bout of depression that seems to arrive for no reason other than to tell me, *"And you thought you were getting better."* This bout holds on tight, a million rubber bands looped all around me, forcing me to work against the tension with every movement, every breath. When I muster enough energy to get out of bed, I sit in my apartment and stare out the window. Each morning, an old man tills a small patch of farmland that wraps around the edge of my building. He tends to his slumbering crops with creaky ease, the ritual ingrained into his body but made harder with age. He steadies himself before each slow kneel to the earth, a puff of hot, white breath condensing in the frigid Baltic air. He roots around in the soil for an offending weed and, with a swift yank, pulls a tangle of roots out of the ground and tosses the intruder into a basket. Then he puts one ungloved hand on the ground, purses his lips, and hoists himself into an arthritic crouch. He straightens up slowly, one vertebra at a time, and scans the soil for another weed to pull. *How familiar the process of sowing seeds must feel,* I think. *How foreign it must be to harvest in a changed body.*

The story doesn't end on the Balkan coast, when Ross and I take an impromptu drive to Bosnia. To our right, the Adriatic Sea glistens in the late-morning sunlight. To the left, endless rocky mountains stand speckled with plots of olive trees, citrus orchards, and vineyards. Around every winding corner, steeples peek out from rocky crags, welcoming us to small towns built into the sides of stone mountains. I roll down my window and stick my arm out to feel the cold, seaside air, letting the force of the wind move my open hand like the waves of the sea beside me.

Before we hit the border, Ross pulls over on the side of the road and we buy a bag of clementines and a little olive oil from a roadside stand. I peel clementine after clementine, filling the rental car with the scent of citrus as we hit the Bosnian countryside just as the sun begins to set. A forest fire in the distance casts a pink, smoky hue on the landscape, and the eerie stillness of the area creeps into the car. It is impossible to tell if the abandoned, pockmarked buildings around us are a casualty of human negligence or of human brutality. Only the occasional steady stream of smoke coming from a chimney tells us the little towns we pass through hold a bit of life.

A thick darkness descends as we climb a series of switchbacks. Ross grips the transmission with white knuckles at each hairpin turn, willing the clutch to shift into gear on the single-lane, cliffside road. It would be so easy for us to stall, to lose control. To roll backwards. To fall.

Even if we survive the drop, we would likely freeze to death. Perhaps it was flippant to come here the way we did, without a plan, without thought. But isn't that how it always goes? One little choice, so small and insignificant at first, ultimately leading you to the last place you ever thought you'd be?

The story doesn't end in Prague, when the rubber bands—for no obvious reason—seem to snap all at once. In one clarifying, unremarkable moment, the room simply brightens. The depression lifts and the rubber bands fall away. The moment doesn't announce itself. There is no fanfare, no ceremony. A nano-glimmer of light simply exists where it didn't before. And that is that. There's nothing more to it, other than the sun shining through my apartment window and I am standing in my underwear when it happens. I wonder if this time it will stick. I wonder if this time I can trust it. I wonder if this wondering, this questioning, will ever end.

The story doesn't end in Portugal, when a gentle breeze carrying sea mist whirls up the cobblestoned street of Rua Possidónio da Silva and tickles my nose as I take a long walk one Sunday. Every day seems like laundry day in Lisbon, with homes displaying a clothesline just outside the front door. I wander by one dwelling with half a dozen pairs of extra-large, robin-egg-blue panties swishing in the wind. I giggle at the thought of hanging your underwear on the street for everyone to see. It strikes me as a bold announcement of humanity, and I wonder if people here were kinder to one another, knowing what's hidden underneath.

The story doesn't end in Mexico City, when my first *taco al pastor* hits my tongue. Thin, crispy bits of pork shaved off a thick *trompo* spiced the color of flames mingle on my palate with soft-yet-hearty masa, tangy sweet pineapple, sharp onion, and grassy cilantro. I devour four tacos in less than a minute.

"I take it we're ordering more?" Ross says, downing his last sip of beer.

"Uh huh," I grunt, grease dribbling down my chin.

Ross raises an empty beer and catches the eye of the man tending to his trompo. "Dos cervezas y cuatro tacos más, por favor."

The al pastor master grins, nods, and slaps a tortilla on his grill.

The story doesn't end when I step out of the airport in Vancouver, Canada and walk into the arms of an old friend. I come to Canada unexpectedly, after my business partner tells me she bought a bar and wants to buy me out and move the bakery into the bar's basement. With the bakery's lease expiring, I choose to take a sabbatical from Remote Year and stay in North America in case I need to fly back to New York to deal with what has become a bitter negotiation. I fight to get what my half was worth, but in the end I cave and sell to her for all of $25,000. Mere pittance. A bailout.

Under the Canadian sky, the smell of pine trees takes me back to the mountains my father and I spent so many afternoons exploring, and I know I can't fight anymore. My heart can't fight anymore. When I put black ink to the sale contract, I push so hard I tear a hole in the page.

The story doesn't end in Buenos Aires, on my last call with Alan. Facing my return to New York, I schedule an appointment with him to work through any lingering fear of going back to my old life. But by the time we got on the phone, and he asks me "so what are we working on today?" I find I am steady. I know I will grieve the loss of traveling, and I will let myself feel it deep. I also know I was not born to wander endlessly. It is time, finally, to focus. It is time to turn the compass toward home.

The story doesn't end in Uruguay, on the banks of the River Plate, in the last moments of my year-long trip around the world. I come here alone, after saying goodbye to Remote Year, to spend a few days by myself on a farm in the small town of Colonia before heading back to New York. When I arrive at my guesthouse, I am greeted by a sandy-red sheepdog named Negroni and the owner of the farmstead who brings me a boule of homemade sourdough bread and honey-orange jam. For three days I do nothing but sip coffee, eat sourdough, and read, surrounded by silent, green farmland. Negroni joins me at all hours of the day, sitting by my feet in the morning and sleeping outside my door at night.

One day, when my body begins to ache from sitting, I take a walk and let Negroni lead the way. She guides me away from the farm, down the main country road, and to a small, dirt path flanked by golden wheat and tall trees blocking the late-afternoon sun. Negroni disappears underneath a wired fence and frolics through the wheat, her red coat bounding above the straw horizon. I call for her and she comes running back, and we continue walking until the farmland falls away and the sky opens up and the ocean appears. I stand in the middle of the road, Negroni at my side, and stare at the distant water.

How far I came to arrive at the edge of Earth, to the edges of myself.

A surge of what can only be described as wild joy rises within me and I run. I run down the dusty dirt road, through a flock of squawking geese, and to the sandy bank. I pull off my shoes and socks, throw them under a tree, and dunk my feet in the water. It is August in Uruguay, winter. The water is frigid and, and as the sun begins to set, the air turns crisp. But I am warmed by the pulse of pure peace and a deep knowing that all of the choices and all of the side effects and all of the questions somehow led me here.

After a while, Negroni nudges me with her wet nose and howls at the sun hanging just above the horizon, telling me it is time to go. I want to stay in this place and wait for the sun to set, to hold onto this feeling as long as I can. Negroni whimpers and paws at my feet until she sees me slip my socks over my sandy feet. My shoes are half of what they were before the year started. The toe box is now peeled away from purple mesh, and the shoelaces no longer stay tied without a double knot. The insoles have long been removed, thrown out after I tried to dry them with a hairdryer in Argentina and inadvertently melted them into a warped mass. Now, all that separates me from the earth is a slim strip of worn rubber. But no matter. They need to stay with me for only a few more days.

I dust myself off and leave shoe prints in the sand as I walk back to the dirt road. As I turn away from the beach, a snarling wild dog runs out of a shack and sends a few geese scampering away in a burst of feathered chaos. My heart leaps into my throat as Negroni darts past me, barking and growling at the dog until it flees back into the shack. Then she circles around me and chases the geese, signaling that the danger is gone and there is no need to worry. I pull back my shoulders, stand tall, walk. My sandy feet crunch inside my shoes and I feel a shoelace slap against my ankle. When I bend down to lace it, I catch a brilliant splash of pink and orange lighting up the sky behind me. I burst alive again on that road, remembering the best part of the sunset happens after the sun falls behind the horizon, when all you're left with is a few moments to breathe in the color of the day before it fades to black. So often, we've already turned our back.

The story doesn't end in New York, as I take the stairs down to Dolores's apartment. The hallway smells of sauerkraut and bratwurst, just as it did a year before. I knock on the door, hear a faint bark. A chain rattles and a dead bolt clunks and the door creaks open. Dolores peers through the crack of the door. Below her, a snout appears.

"Ooooohhhh! What a surprise!" Dolores squeals. "Buffy, look who's here! Come in!" She ushers me through the door and I turn my attention to Buffy, waiting for her to paw at my shins and whine and jump at me like she used to do every time I came home from the bakery.

But Buffy just stands there and looks at me with indifference. After a few moments she tucks her head, walks to my feet, and gives them a sniff. She moves with tender steps, her fur scraggly, her eyes cloudier than I remember. She meets my eyes as I crouch down to her. Her little tail wags gently, and she lets me scratch her ear. She gives me a gentle lick on the nose, but as Dolores shuffles past me and moves toward the couch, Buffy's head follows her. When Dolores sits down, Buffy pulls away from me, goes to the old woman, and rests at her feet. Buffy stares at me from across the room, a content look on her face that seems to say, "You can go now. We are all settled here."

In that moment, I know I am done with New York. For good.

The story doesn't end in Reno, on an overstuffed chair, a year into writing this book. I am stuck at a juncture between memory and truth, unsure of where to take a narrative thread or how best to tell it. My mother comes into the room, a cloudy Ziploc bag of cassette tapes hanging from her hands.

"I just found these buried in the closet," she tells me. "They're recordings of your father, when he was your age, working with a spiritual counselor kind of like Alan. The woman's name was Mary. I don't know what's on them, but I know they were important to him. I've never listened to them, but it's interesting that they showed up now."

She hands me the tapes, gives me a hug, and heads off to work.

I find an old cassette tape player in the back of a drawer, in between a first-generation Game Boy and a puzzle. I reach into the bag and pick a tape labeled "Warren 5/22/1977," and press play. The song "Call on Me" by Chicago comes blasting through the cassette player's scratchy speakers. Someone had recorded the radio over his session, but somehow the musical recording didn't quite stick and buried underneath the song was my father's thirty-year-old voice. His tone is not as gruff as I remember, but, still, it is him.

The song plays while Mary and my father gurgle behind it.

"Then came a change/When I said I would soon be leavin' you."

I put my ear to the speaker, trying to tune out the music, and listen for clear words.

Mary's voice comes through. "The scientific community has found that everything in the universe has energy, and energy cannot be destroyed. It has to go someplace . . . "

"Nothin' else to do," the song continues.

" . . . everything has energy: plants, rocks, the sun, you, me."

"Please remember I never lose the thought of you."

" . . . and when those energies come and trigger your energies . . . "

"I love you, you know I do."

" . . . the quality of that moment . . . "

Mary's voice fades away and the remainder of the tape is nothing but music—Brian Auger, Joni Mitchell, Jefferson Starship. I flip the tape to side B, expecting more of the same, but instead my father's voice comes booming through: "How about the effects of the affair?"

He is preoccupied with a drunken one-night stand after he returned from fighting in the Vietnam War and before he met my mother.

"Within each day," Mary says, "make sure you get through it with honesty."

Their voices gurgle to a halt. I eject the tape, throw it aside, and take another from the bag, dated 4/12/78. On side A, it's Jesus Christ Superstar and Elton John. On side B, it's my father recounting a vacation to the Redwoods. He got an eighteen-ounce steak with all the trimmings, peas and carrots and potatoes and pie, all for seven dollars, and then made love to a woman named Lorraine in a field full of daisies.

On the next tape, he and Lorraine have broken up.

"I'm still down here, fighting against reality," he says. He is thirty-two now, the same age as me, driving semi-trucks back and forth across the country in order to make a living. He doesn't know that within a year he will meet my mother and a few years after that I will come along. It is odd to listen to my father talk about his world before I existed, to hear a softness in his voice as he grapples with the harsh truths of living. I can hear him swing back and forth between light and dark, finding morsels of his humanity in the presence of nature or while driving on the open road, only to be hammered down by his own intensity that seems to destroy anything he touches.

"You are a spiritual being in a human body," Mary tells him. "The Earth will always show you what you need to learn."

"That's the part that's so goddamn difficult to handle," my father says. "Sometimes I'll go into a store and I just want to get what I'm there for. I need to buy an ice cream cone or a hamburger or something, and it's like my intensity—it's like people don't want to be around me." My father's typically booming voice softens with the twinge of shame. "But then sometimes I make a joke or I smile . . . "

"And they relax," Mary says. "There is a knowing, Warren, that everybody is one. Let's say we are all ice cubes. If we were to dissolve, we would just go back into a giant puddle. You wouldn't know who was what or when or where or what color. Because we are all one."

"And that's the energy source?" my father asks.

"That's the energy source. And if there's a bad energy over here, we cannot throw it away or turn our back on it. That's the one we have to heal. Because if there is one little bit of impurity in the water, the whole puddle becomes impure. All you have to understand, Warren, is that you are still a student. You are still working on this assignment. This Earth is not our home. It is our school."

There are a dozen of these tapes, with just as many hours of recordings to sift through. I dump out all the tapes on the carpet and arrange them in chronological order, from 1977 to 1989. In the middle of the pack, a date stands out: February 1, 1986. The day I was born.

I load the tape and press play.

My father's voice: "Testing one, two, three, four. A cow jumped over the moon. Don't know what this is going to sound like."

Mumbled voices emerge. A heart monitor beeps quick with life. Metal tools clink. A high-pitched wail. Me.

At the sound of my first cry, I start to sob. The experience of listening to my birth, and my father's place in it all, is surreal. My mother is unconscious on the table, given general anesthesia for an emergency C-section when the doctor discovered I had wrapped the umbilical cord around my neck three times. I was prepping to hang myself upon exit, apparently, and my father would need to be the one to cradle me.

The nurses wipe me off and place me in my father's arms. "She's awful quiet," he says. "Are they supposed to sleep like this right away?"

"It's not really a true sleep," the doctor says. "She's okay."

"I never thought I'd get married, let alone have children . . . " My father trails off.

"The situation gets heavier all the time, doesn't it?" the doctor says.

My father goes quiet. The situation is now six pounds, thirteen ounces heavier in his arms. Nurses mill about around him. A rusty wheel squeaks. After a few minutes, my father speaks again, his voice wavering.

"What about her eyes, doc? Are her eyes okay? I had a bad dream that she was born without eyes."

The doctor stops whatever he is doing, curious about why my father would mention such a thing. I hear his footsteps come closer to my father and stop, the two men standing next to each other, hovering over me. The doctor's scrubs rustle as he gives me a once-over. Through thirty-two years of time, I can feel my father holding his breath, holding me.

"Don't worry," the doctor says. "See how her pupils open and close? It means she's okay. She can see, Warren. She can see the light."

afterword

It has been six years since I took my last antidepressant and still, I am searching for the ending. Some part of me can't stop digging back through time, looking for the moment when I can say, for certain, that the tendrils of depression, antidepressants, and antidepressant withdrawal no longer intertwine with what I know to be true about myself, my experiences, my life. But I keep coming up short.

All I know for sure was that I was a minor when the drugs were first prescribed to me. No one forced the drugs down my throat each morning, but through my fifteen-year-old eyes, I had little choice in the matter and no reason to question the adults around me. Any frame of reference for who I was without drugs existed before my father died, when I was a child. The world through antidepressants was all I knew and I lived in it, without question, until I was thirty. I tell you this not to place blame, but because I think it's important to understand that at the time the decision was made to medicate me, no one could have predicted the outcome.

The same can be said about the rash method in which I was pulled off the antidepressants. I took Dr. Chin's advice and stopped the Effexor XR cold turkey because she was the expert and I assumed she was fully informed on the subject. I didn't do my own research. Even if I had, there wouldn't have been much to find. Despite years of patient suffering, research into antidepressant withdrawal has been a low priority for doctors and psychiatrists. The first systematic review of antidepressant withdrawal did not even exist until 2015[1], a full twenty-eight years after Prozac was first released to the public in 1987.

---

1   Giovanni A. Fava et al., "Withdrawal Symptoms after Selective Serotonin Reuptake Inhibitor Discontinuation," *Psychotherapy and Psychosomatics* 84 (Febraury 2015): 72–81.

Finally, in 2019, the first comprehensive systematic analysis of antidepressant withdrawal found that more than half of people coming off antidepressants experience withdrawal symptoms, and half of those—like me—experience severe withdrawal.[2] A separate study of those suffering from antidepressant-associated post-acute withdrawal syndrome (PAWS) found that participants experienced withdrawal symptoms for an average of thirty-seven months, with 81 percent of participants reporting suicidality as a direct effect of their withdrawal symptoms.[3]

To make matters more complicated, withdrawal symptoms are often confused with the relapse (or return) of the original diagnoses or are considered an emergence of a new mental disorder. This confusion can lead to misdiagnosis and medicalization for psychiatric disorders that don't actually exist in the patient. In the wrong hands, my symptoms could have garnered a diagnosis for everything from bipolar disorder to psychosis to schizophrenia, all of which would have resulted in serious pharmaceutical intervention. If these drugs were easy to manage with few side effects, perhaps this misdiagnosis wouldn't be an egregious oversight. But psychiatric diagnosis changes lives, and psychiatric drugs are powerful substances that should not be given or taken away without serious consideration of both short *and* long-term effects. Remember, it only takes five minutes to prescribe a psychiatric drug, but it can take years to get off them.

The good news is that research now shows that the best way to get off antidepressants and antianxiety drugs is through hyperbolic tapering, a dose reduction method that calls for smaller and smaller decreases, especially near the end of a taper. It's not a perfect strategy, but it is more likely to mitigate serious, long-term withdrawal symptoms.[4] [5] Despite the existence of this research, though, countless people around the world are still being harmed by rushed and arcane tapers. To ensure that the message of this book is clear, let me state it plainly: Never abruptly stop taking psychiatric drugs, even at

2   James Davies and John Read, "A Systematic Review into the Incidence, Severity and Duration of Antidepressant Withdrawal Effects," *Addictive Behaviors* 97 (August 2019):111–21.

3   Michael P. Hengartner et al., "Protracted Withdrawal Syndrome after Stopping Antidepressants," *Therapeutic Advances in Psychopharmacology* 10 (December 2020).

4   Mark A. Horowitz and David Taylor, "Tapering of SSRI Treatment to Mitigate Withdrawal Symptoms," *The Lancet Psychiatry* 6, no. 6 (June 2019): 538–46.

5   Adele Framer, "What I Have Learnt from Helping Thousands of People Taper Off Psychotropic Medications," *Therapeutic Advances in Psychopharmacology* 11 (January 2021).

low or "therapeutic" doses. Had I known about hyperbolic tapering, it's likely this book would never have needed to be written.

Of course, I didn't know what I didn't know. As a result, the decision to both go on antidepressants at fifteen and get off them at thirty continues to reverberate with curious consequences. The debilitating aspects of withdrawal—the unrelenting mood swings, the sensory overload, the murderous, intrusive thoughts—are long gone. Other smaller reminders remain. The nodular vasculitis in my limbs exists in a state of fragile dormancy. Existential stress flares it up, and when dark patches and tender bumps appear, I know something in my life needs serious readjusting.

Noise sensitivity also continues to plague me, though I am proud to announce I no longer turn gray at the sound of a leaf blower. I did, however, move from a maple-tree-lined street to the desert, where there are fewer leaves to blow. As Alan once said, sometimes instead of trying to make where you are more tolerable, you need to take control and find a more tolerable place. Moving to a quiet home, in addition to a pair of custom-made earplugs, has allowed me to both live in peace and to better handle noise when it does come around, since my nervous system isn't on high alert all the time.

The intangible effects of withdrawal, though, continue to haunt me. Most days I am lost in *what if.* What if I'd never been put on the drugs in the first place? How would my life be different? Would it be different? Would I have wanted the life I lived, or would I have still found myself at a window, contemplating the body's rate of fall?

Think about it: My father's sudden death and my subsequent introduction to the hazy world of antidepressants dropped me into an alternate reality at a time when I was forming the foundation of my identity. I was told there was something wrong with my mind and the only "fix" was medication. I made every decision from that moment on through the lens of brokenness. I went through puberty under the influence of antidepressants and came out the other side with shapely hips and the assumption that my brain and body had developed into the adult I was always meant to be. In a sense, it didn't matter what college I went to or what job I got or where I lived. I was going to be broken no matter what. Broken was not my fault, but it was my default. Thriving was out of the question, happiness nothing more than a fairy-tale construct. So I aimed to create a tolerable life because a tolerable life built on a broken foundation was the best I believed I could hope for.

A tolerable existence is found on the path of least resistance, where decisions are made out of obligation, not meaning. There isn't much forethought on this path, I find. It's all about defaulting to the situation that takes the least amount of energy. Therefore, I didn't invest in lasting relationships. I blamed my disinterest on introversion, but that's just the story I told myself. The truth is waiting to die went by faster when I was alone than it did when I was with other people. Even though I spent most of my free time by myself, I never bothered to learn anything new or keep up the skills I already had. I didn't spend time thinking about savings or IRAs or wondering what I was going to do with myself when the bakery closed. I figured the next thing would emerge on the path and I'd do it until it was over. And the next and the next and the next until I ran out of future all together. On a basic level, that's the definition of life. But it never occurred to me to stack the deck in my favor. Extending extra effort is not part of the path of least resistance. I didn't want a future, so why plan for one?

Now I want it all. I want all the futures I never had. I want the life I chose and the ones I didn't. I want to know a timeline in which I'd never been medicated and one where my father never died. I want a timeline of stable love and another of untethered freedom. I want to know who I'd be if I'd taken over the family business, stayed in New York, or chosen a different college. I want a timeline on a stretch of farmland, spending my days writing and tending to chickens. I want a timeline of running marathons, and another still in silence. I want endless pleasure and the structure of discipline. I want to feel it all, be it all. I want to stay and leave and come back again, weaving in and out from one timeline to another, over and over until I've lived each choice and determined for sure that this is the one.

But it is exhausting to live in worlds that don't exist, and I am tiring from wading back through time. I have already chosen a life. This one. Though all the other timelines will continue to turn around me, reminding me of who I could have been, maybe the truth is there is no one right choice. Maybe every choice is neutral, the idea of "good" or "bad" nothing more than personal projection. Maybe the work isn't about learning to make the "right" choice but learning to let go of all the ones never made. This is the only truth. Any other life, any other timeline, is little more than fiction.

As for the characters who wove in and out of my life during this year, though they all crossed my path independently, together, they saved my life. Ben spent a few more years in Cambodia before moving on to Vietnam and eventually settling back in the States. Martin left Thailand and moved to the blue waters of Indonesia, where he met someone and created the true love of his life—his daughter. Ross never stayed still after Remote Year and is meandering from place to place, often falling off the grid for months at a time while seeking cozy Central American towns in which to surf and work. Wilson's colorful shipping container hostel is still open and operating in Sekinchan, and Nik is thriving as the founder and content creator of a Malaysian pop-culture media company.

Buffy lived out the rest of her sixteen years with Dolores, who, as of this writing, is still kicking ass at ninety-one. She has continued the tradition of dog-sitting other pups in the building and is in high demand, currently juggling two canines from two different families.

After seeing the impact Alan's work had on me, my mother sold the collection agency she ran for forty years and became a student of Alan and his self-compassion modality. She now uses the methodology to help people all over the world. We also live fifteen minutes away from each other, and there has been no greater gift in my adult life than getting to be so close to my mother, my best friend.

All this to say that the woman who stood at her thirtieth-story window—I barely recognize her. I can't tell you when she began to fade from my recognition. But at some point over the past five years, the spotlight of my mind shifted from her suffering and began shining on little moments where I seem to awaken from the darkness and blink alive. That's the trouble with healing. It begins with such subtlety that it's easy to miss. Day-to-day improvements are but a single nail hammered into wood, barely noticeable until hundreds and thousands of nails work together to hold a stable shape. But each nail is an ode to the possibility of joy and lightness and an ease so all-encompassing that when I look back, my first thought does not fall on the darkness. Instead, I remember the light.

Maybe the story doesn't ever really end. Maybe the focus simply shifts, the blurry end of one story just the beginning of another.

Brooke Siem
March 2022

acknowledgments

From conception to publishing date, *May Cause Side Effects* took 1874 days to complete. I'd like to thank the following people, places, and things—in no particular order—for ushering me along the brutal and beautiful process of book writing:

Laura Munson, writer extraordinaire and founder of Haven Writing Retreats, who cracked open my manuscript and brought it to life. The Nevada Arts Council for their grant that helped fund my time at Haven. Beth Davey, my literary agent, who did the impossible and sold a book about antidepressant withdrawal during a global pandemic. Jeff Speich and Valerie Killeen at Central Recovery Press. Thank you for believing in me. Here's hoping it pays off! Matt O'Brien, your edits made this book far better. I'm sorry I still don't know how to use hyphens correctly. Blue Diamond Smoked Almonds for fueling my morning writing sessions since 2017. Nova Robinson, for loaning me her Seattle apartment and pumping me with champagne at the conclusion of my first legitimate draft. Ann Maynard of Command+Z Content, who edited my first (terrible) 20,000 words and encouraged me to keep going. Joe Johnston and Alpheus Chan, for knowing me long enough to buy me dinner and let me word vomit all over them whenever the starving artist life gets hard. Sid Meier's Civilization 6. Every one of The Tots—you all were part of the greatest learning experience of my life. Thank you for accepting me even when I was being a jerk. Mack's Silicone Earplugs—from drowning out the sounds of college dorms to quieting the screams of toddlers on international flights, you might be the most valuable object in my life. The Binders. Every evening out at a good-for-Reno restaurant with Zachary Shea. Long walks with Atchariya

Fletcher. I miss you. Dr. Tracy Protell and her psychiatric notes on later drafts. Johann Hari for donating his time to help this little writerling off the ground. Tiffany Schegg, Radhika Siddharthan, Mary Rose Walker, and Taylor Calderone—your recollections of our childhood have helped me piece myself together as an adult. I'm so glad we're still in each other's lives. Justin Alger, you. You have been with me for every one of these 1874 days, never wavering despite the hurricanes it created. Your love has turned me into a better human.

Lastly, my mother, Dee. You once told me that every morning, you surround me with a beam of white light in your mind's eye. As I've gotten older and learned to harness the power of gratitude, it is you who comes to my mind each day. Thank you for picking up the phone every single time, for helping me chase moonshots like opening a bakery and writing a book, and for eschewing parental norms and treating me like a partner rather than a perpetual child. Your wisdom inspired the underlying themes of this book, and I'm so glad I get to share it with the world.

Printed in the USA
CPSIA information can be obtained
at www.ICGtesting.com
JSHW080541230324
59758JS00001B/21